KEY NOTES ON

Plastic Sur

ADRIAN M. RICHARDS
MSc FRCS (Plast.)
Consultant Plastic Surgeon
Stoke Mandeville NHS Trust
Aylesbury
Buckinghamshire
United Kingdom

FOREWORD BY

PROFESSOR IAN T. JACKSON
Director of Craniofacial and Reconstructive Surgery
Providence Hospital
Michigan
USA

Blackwell
Science

a Blackwell Publishing Company
Editorial Offices:
Osney Mead, Oxford OX2 0EL, UK
Tel: +44 (0)1865 206206
Blackwell Science, Inc., 350 Main Street, Malden, MA 02148-5018, USA
Tel: +1 781 388 8250
Blackwell Science Asia Pty, 54 University Street, Carlton, Victoria 3053, Australia
Tel: +61 (0)3 9347 0300
Blackwell Wissenschafts Verlag, Kurfürstendamm 57, 10707 Berlin, Germany
Tel: +49 (0)30 32 79 060

First published 2002

2 2007

Library of Congress Cataloging-in-Publication Data

Richards, Adrian M. Key notes on plastic surgery/Adrian M. Richards; foreword by Ian Jackson.
p. cm.
Includes index.
ISBN 978-0-6320-5668-2 (pbk.)
1. Surgery, Plastic—Handbooks, manuals etc. I. Title.
[DNLM: 1. Surgery, Plastic WO 600 R514k 2001]
617.9′5—dc21

ISBN 978-0-6320-5668-2

A catalogue record for this title is available from the British Library

Set in 9.5 on 12pt Galliard by Graphicraft Limited, Hong Kong
Printed and bound in Singapore by Utopia Press Pte Ltd

For further information on Blackwell Science, visit our website:
www.blackwell-science.com

Contents

Foreword

I am particularly critical of the large numbers of plastic surgery textbooks being produced by well-known and little-known companies, and authored by well-known and little-known authors. The latter range from dermatologists through oral surgeons to ear, nose and throat surgeons and plastic surgeons. One wonders why these books are ever written, why they are ever published, and especially why anyone would ever want to buy them. When *Key Notes on Plastic Surgery* was sent to me, my feeling was, 'Oh, no, not another useless, general plastic surgery textbook'. How wrong I was. This is a plastic surgery textbook with a difference. The difference is that it is not a large book, it is not filled with unnecessary padding and photographs, be they good or awful. This contains only the meat without all the unnecessary trimmings. It is not filled with references which are designed to make the reader think that the author has researched all of them (most of these references are never used except in the production of yet another chapter or yet another book).

This book has a definite purpose and, as such, it truly fills a void in plastic surgery. It is a distillation of plastic surgery and contains only the significant facts laid out in a clear fashion with economy of words—a rare feature of the modern textbook! This being so, it will be used clinically by a multitude of trainees and also by fully fledged plastic surgeons. I can also see it being consulted prior to surgery and certainly prior to examinations. It might, on occasion, even find its way into the operating room! I especially appreciate the economy of words, it makes for easier registration of facts.

Adrian Richards is to be congratulated on seeing the need for such a book and to have set it out in such a clear and informative fashion. I heartily recommend it to those in training, and to those who are somewhat older and want to quickly review techniques and brush up on those which have stood the test of time. I have a feeling that this will be the first of many editions, and it will become a significant textbook in the training of plastic surgeons in the UK and Europe, and, hopefully, given the proper exposure, in the United States. I consider it an honour, and certainly it has been a pleasure, to be invited to write this foreword.

Ian T. Jackson, MD

Preface

When preparing for the plastic surgical exam at the end of my training, I bought almost every plastic surgical text on the market in the hope that this would guarantee success. I found it difficult and time consuming to extract information from the larger texts and rued the lack of a short and succinct book to help me with my studies. This book aims to provide the reader with a sturdy scaffold of plastic surgical knowledge, which can then be supplemented from other sources. I hope that it will be useful to plastic surgeons of all levels the world over; if it makes exam preparation any less frustrating it will have served its purpose.

Adrian M. Richards

Dedication

To the memory of my mother, Jill Lovesey

To my father, David

To my wife, Helena, and my children, Josie, Ciara and Alfie

Acknowledgements

I would like to thank my many trainers and mentors for their teaching, advice and inspiration, particularly Michael Klaassen, Professor Gus McGrouther, Robert McDowall, John Hobby, Richard Cole, Michael Cadier, Tim Goodacre, David Coleman, Steven Wall, Henk Giele, Graham Southwick, Simon Donahoe, Morris Ritz, Damien Ireland, Anthony Berger and Steven Tham.

I have appreciated the advice and support of my fellow trainees Michael Tyler, David Johnson and Andrew Pay, who have given me valuable advice while preparing the book. Paul Cohen, David Lam, Emma Hormbrey and Tom MacLeod spent many hours proofreading the text for which I am grateful. I would also like to thank Mr Parkhouse for reviewing the manuscript in its early stages. I am indebted to Stuart Taylor, Rosie Hayden, Debbie Maizels, Rupal Malde, and all those at Blackwell Science for their help in getting the book to print. Finally I would like to thank my wife, Helena, for her patience and support.

Abbreviations

ABPI	ankle brachial pressure indices
ADM	abductor digiti minimi
AER	apical ectodermal ridge
AFX	atypical fibroxanthoma
AK	actinic keratosis
ALM	acral lentiginous melanoma
AP	anteroposterior
APB	abductor pollicis brevis
APL	abductor pollicis longus
ARDS	adult respiratory distress syndrome
ASA	American Society of Anesthesiologists
AVA	arteriovenous anastomosis
AVM	arteriovenous malformation
AVN	avascular necrosis
BAPS	British Association of Plastic Surgeons
BCC	basal cell carcinoma
BEAM	bulbar elongation and anastomotic meatoplasty
BMP	bone morphogenic protein
BOA	British Orthopaedic Association
BP	blood pressure
BSA	body surface area
BXO	balinitis xerotica obliterans
CL	cleft lip
CMCJ	carpometacarpal joint
CMF	cisplatin, melphalan, 5-fluouracil
CO	carbon monoxide
CP	cleft palate
CT	computed tomography
DBD	dermolytic bullous dermatitis
DCIA	deep circumflex iliac artery
DCIS	ductal carcinoma *in situ*
DEC	diethylcarbamazepine
DFSP	dermatofibrosarcoma protuberans
DIC	disseminated intravascular coagulation
DIEA	deep inferior epigastric artery
DIEP	deep inferior epigastric perforator (flap)
DIPJ	distal interphalangeal joint
DISI	dorsal intercalated segment instability
DOPA	dihydroxyphenylalanine

DOT	double-opposing tab
ECRB	extensor carpi radialis brevis
ECRL	extensor carpi radialis longus
ECU	extensor carpi ulnaris
EDC	extensor digitorum communis
EDM	extensor digiti minimi
EHL	extensor hallucis longus
EIP	extensor indicis proprius
ELND	elective lymph node dissection
EMG	electromyograph
EPB	extensor pollicis brevis
EPL	extensor pollicis longus
ESR	erythrocyte sedimentation rate
FBC	full blood count
FCR	flexor carpi radialis
FCU	flexor carpi ulnaris
FDA	Food and Drug Administration
FDM	flexor digiti minimi
FDP	flexor digitorum profundus
FDS	flexor digitorum superficialis
FGF	fibroblast growth factor
FNA	fine needle aspiration
FPB	flexor pollicis brevis
FPL	flexor pollicis longus
GAG	glycosaminoglycan
GHN	giant hairy naevus
GI	gastro-intestinal
Hb	haemoglobin
HIV	human immunodeficiency virus
HLA	human leucocyte antigen
HPV	human papilloma virus
ICD	intercanthal distance
ICP	intercranial pressure
IDDM	insulin dependent diabetes mellitus
IF	interferon
IL	interleukin
IOP	interorbital distance
IPJ	interphalangeal joint
IPPV	intermittent positive pressure ventilation
IVP	intravenous pyelogram
KA	keratoacanthoma
LA	local anaesthesia
LASER	light amplification by stimulated emission of radiation
LCIS	lobular carcinoma *in situ*
LM	lentigo maligna

LME	line of maximum extensibility
LMM	lentigo maligna melanoma
MAGPI	meatal advancement and glanuloplasty incorporated
MCPJ	metacarpophalangeal joint
MFH	malignant fibrous histiocytoma
MHC	major histocompatibility complex
MM	malignant melanoma
MRC	Medical Research Council
MRI	magnetic resonance imaging
mRNA	messenger ribonucleic acid
MRSA	methicillin resistant *Staphylococcus aureus*
MSG	Melanoma Study Group
MSH	melanocyte-stimulating hormone
MUM	monosodium urate monohydrate
NAC	nipple areolar complex
NK	natural killer (cell)
NSAID	non-steroidal anti-inflammatory drug
OA	osteoarthritis
OM	occipital mental
OPG	orthopantomogram
OR&IF	open reduction and internal fixation
PA	posteroanterior
PB	peroneus brevis
PCR	polymerase chain reaction
PDGF	platelet-derived growth factor
PDS	polydioxanone suture
PE	pulmonary embolus
PIPJ	proximal interphalangeal joint
PL	peroneus longus
PL	palmaris longus
PT	peroneus tertius
PT	pronator teres
PTFE	polytetrafluoroethylene
RA	retinoic acid
RA	rheumatoid arthritis
RCL	radial collateral ligament
RFF	radial-forearm flap
ROOF	retro-orbicularis oculi fat (pad)
RSD	reflex sympathetic dystrophy
RSTL	relaxed skin tension line
RT-PCR	reverse transcriptase-polymerase chain reaction
S-GAP	superior gluteal artery perforator (flap)
SCC	squamous cell carcinoma
SCIA	superficial circumflex iliac artery
SLE	systemic lupus erythematosus

SLL	scapholunate ligament
SLAC	scapholunate advanced collapse
SMAS	superficial musculoaponeurotic system
SMR	submucous resection
SNAC	scaphoid nonunion advanced collapse
SOOF	suborbicularis oculi fat (pad)
SSG	split-skin graft
SSM	superficial spreading melanoma
TBSA	total body surface area
TCA	trichloroacetic acid
TFCC	triangular fibrocartilagenous complex
TFL	tensor fascia lata
TGF	transforming growth factor
TLND	therapeutic lymph node dissection
TMJ	temporomandibular joint
TMN	tumour, metastases, nodes
TNF	tumour necrosis factor
t-PA	tissue plasminogen activator
TPN	total parental nutrition
TRAM	transverse rectus abdominis muscle
UAL	ultrasonic assisted liposuction
UCL	ulnar collateral ligament
UV	ultraviolet
VAC	vacuum-assisted closure
VCF	velocardiofacial (syndrome)
VISI	volar intercalated segment instability
VPI	velopharyngeal incompetence
VRAM	vertical rectus abdominis myocutaneous (flap)
WLE	wide local excision
XP	xeroderma pigmentosa
ZF	zygomaticofrontal

1

General principles

Structure and function of the skin

The functions of the skin include:

1 Physical protection
2 Protection against UV light
3 Protection against microbiological invasion
4 Prevention of fluid loss
5 Regulation of body temperature
6 Sensation
7 Immunological surveillance.

The epidermis

- The epidermis is composed of stratified squamous epithelium.
- It is derived from ectoderm.
- Epidermal cells undergo keratinization in which their cytoplasm is replaced with keratin as the cell dies and becomes more superficial.

The epidermis is composed of the following five layers, from deep to superficial.

1 Stratum germinativum

- This is also known as the basal layer.
- The cells within this layer have cytoplasmic projections, which firmly link them to the underlying basal lamina.

- This is the only actively proliferating layer of skin.
- The stratum germinativum contains melanocytes.

2 Stratum spinosum
- The stratum spinosum is also known as the prickle cell layer.
- This layer contains large keratinocytes which produce keratin.
- The cells within this layer are joined to each other by tonofibrils (prickles).

3 Stratum granulosum
- The stratum granulosum contains mature keratinocytes, which possess cytoplasmic granules of keratohyalin.
- This layer is called the stratum granulosum because of these granules.
- The stratum granulosum is the predominant site of protein synthesis.

4 Stratum lucidum
- This is a clear layer.
- The stratum lucidum is only present in the thick skin of the palms and feet.

5 Stratum corneum
- The stratum corneum contains non-viable keratinized cells.
- The thick cells of this layer protect against trauma.
- The stratum corneum:
  - Insulates against fluid loss
  - Protects against bacterial invasion.
- Sebum produced by the sebaceous glands of the stratum corneum is bactericidal to both streptococci and staphylococci.

Cellular composition of the epidermis
- Keratinocytes are the predominant cell type in the epidermis.
- Langerhans cells form part of the immune system and function as antigen-presenting cells.
- Merkel cells are mechanoreceptors of neural crest origin.
- Melanocytes:
  - Are neural crest derivatives
  - Are usually located in the stratum germinativum
  - Produce melanin, which protects the surrounding skin by absorbing UV light.

The dermis
- The dermis accounts for 95% of the thickness of the skin.
- The papillary dermis is superficial and contains more cells and finer collagen fibres.
- The reticular dermis is deeper and contains fewer cells and coarser collagen fibres.

The dermis is composed of the following.

Collagen fibres

· These fibres are produced by fibroblasts.
· They are responsible for much of the strength of the skin.
· The normal ratio of type 1 to type 3 collagen is 5 : 1.

Elastin fibres

· These are secreted by fibroblasts.
· They are responsible for the elastic recoil of the skin.

Ground substance

· This consists of the glycosaminoglycans (GAGs), hyaluronic acid, dermatan sulfate and chondroitin sulfate.
· GAGs are secreted by fibroblasts and become ground substance when hydrated.

Vascular plexus

· This separates the denser reticular dermis from the overlying papillary dermis.

Skin appendages

The skin contains the following appendages.

Hair follicles

· Each hair is composed of a medulla, cortex and outer cuticle.
· The hair follicle consists of an inner root sheath, derived from the epidermis, and an outer root sheath, derived from the dermis.
· Several sebaceous glands drain into each follicle. Discharge from these glands is aided by the contraction of erector pili muscles.
· Velus hairs are fine and downy.
· Terminal hairs are coarse.
· Hairs are in either the telogen or the anogen phase.
· 75% of hairs are in the anogen (growth) phase at any one time.
· The remaining 25% of hairs are in the telogen (resting) phase.

Eccrine glands

· These sweat glands secrete an odourless hypotonic fluid.
· They are present in all sites of the body.
· Eccrine glands occur more frequently in the eyelids, palms, feet and axilla.

Apocrine glands

· These are located in the axilla and groin.
· They emit a thicker secretion than eccrine glands.
· They are responsible for body odour.
· Hidradenitis suppurativa is an infection of the apocrine glands.

Sebaceous glands

· These are holocrine glands that usually drain into the pilosebaceous unit.

· They drain directly onto the skin in the labia, penis and tarsus (meibomian glands).
· They occur more frequently on the forehead, nose and cheek.
· Sebaceous glands are not the sole cause of so-called sebaceous cysts. These cysts are in fact of epidermal origin and contain all of the substances secreted by the skin (predominantly keratin).
· Some authorities maintain that they should therefore be called epidermoid cysts.

Types of secretion from glands

· Eccrine or merocrine glands secrete opened vesicles via exocytosis.
· Apocrine glands secrete unbroken vesicles which later discharge.
· Holocrine glands secrete whole cells which then disintegrate.

Histological terms

· Acanthosis—hyperplasia of the epithelium.
· Papillomatosis—an increase in the depth of the corrugations at the junction between epidermis and dermis.
· Hyperkeratosis—an increase in the thickness of the keratin layer.
· Parakeratosis—the presence of nucleated cells at the skin surface.

Blood supply to the skin

Anatomy of the circulation

· The blood reaching the skin originates from deep vessels.
· These then feed interconnecting vessels which supply the vascular plexuses of fascia, subcutaneous tissue and skin.

Deep vessels

The deep vessels arise from the aorta and divide to form the main arterial supply to the head, neck, trunk and limbs.

Interconnecting vessels

The interconnecting system is composed of:

· Fasciocutaneous (or septocutaneous) perforating vessels
  · These vessels reach the skin by traversing fascial septae.
  · They provide the main arterial supply to the skin in the limbs.
· Musculocutaneous vessels
  · These vessels reach the skin via direct muscular branches from the deep system.
  · These branches enter muscle bellies and divide into multiple perforating branches, which travel up to the skin.
  · The musculocutaneous system provides the main arterial supply to the skin of the torso.

Vascular plexuses of fascia, subcutaneous tissue and skin

Vascular plexuses of the fascia, subcutaneous tissue and skin are divided into six layers.

1 Subfascial plexus
- A small plexus lying on the undersurface of the fascia.

2 Prefascial plexus
- A larger plexus particularly prominent on the limbs.
- Predominantly supplied by fasciocutaneous vessels.

3 Subcutaneous plexus
- Lies at the level of the superficial fascia.
- Mainly supplied by musculocutaneous vessels.
- Predominant on the torso.

4 Subdermal plexus
- Receives blood from the underlying plexuses.
- The main plexus supplying blood to the skin.
- Represented by dermal bleeding observed in incised skin.

5 Dermal plexus
- Mainly composed of arterioles.
- Plays an important role in thermoregulation.

6 Subepidermal plexus
- Contains small vessels without muscle in their walls.
- Has a predominantly nutritive and thermoregulatory function.

Angiosomes

- An angiosome is a composite block of tissue supplied by a named artery.
- The area of skin supplied by an artery was first studied by Manchot in 1889.
- His work was expanded by Salmon in the early 1930s, and more recently by Taylor and Palmer.
- The anatomical territory of an artery is the area in which the vessel branches ramify before anastomosing with adjacent vessels.
- The dynamic territory of an artery is the area into which staining extends after intravascular infusion of fluorescein.
- The potential territory of an artery is the area that can be included in a flap if it is delayed.
- The vessels that pass between anatomical territories are called choke vessels.

The transverse rectus abdominis muscle (TRAM) flap illustrates the angiosome concept well.

- *Zone 1*
  - This receives musculocutaneous perforators from the deep inferior epigastric artery (DIEA) and is therefore in its anatomical territory.
- *Zones 2 and 3*
  - There is some controversy as to which of the following zones is 2 and which is 3; the numbers of these zones are interchanged in various texts.
  - The portion of skin lateral to zone 1 is in the anatomical territory of the superficial circumflex iliac artery (SCIA). Blood has to travel through a set of choke vessels to reach it from the ipsilateral DIEA.

- The portion of skin on the other side of the linea alba is in the anatomical area of the contralateral DIEA. This area is reliably perfused in a TRAM flap based on the contralateral DIEA and is therefore within its dynamic territory.

- *Zone 4*
  - This lies furthest from the pedicle and is in the anatomical territory of the contralateral SCIA.
  - Blood passing from the flap pedicle to zone 4 has to cross two sets of choke vessels.
  - This portion of the TRAM flap has the worst blood supply and for this reason it is often discarded.

Arterial characteristics

From his detailed anatomical dissections Taylor made the following observations:

1 Vessels usually travel with nerves.
2 Vessels obey the law of equilibrium—if one is small, its neighbour will tend to be large.
3 Vessels travel from fixed to mobile tissue.
4 Vessels have a fixed destination but a varied origin.
5 Vessel size and orientation is a product of growth.

The microcirculation

- Terminal arterioles are present in the reticular dermis and terminate as they enter the capillary network.
- The precapillary sphincter is the last part of the arterial tree containing muscle within its wall. It is under neural control and regulates the blood flow into the capillary network.
- Arteriovenous anastomoses (AVAs) connect the arterioles to the efferent veins.
- Blood flowing through AVAs bypasses the capillary bed and has a thermoregulatory rather than nutritive function.
- AVAs are of two types:
  1 Indirect AVAs are convoluted structures known as glomera and are densely innervated by autonomic nerves.
  2 Direct AVAs are much less convoluted and have a sparser autonomic supply.
- The blood supply to the skin far exceeds its nutritive requirements—much of it bypasses the capillary beds via the AVAs and has a primarily thermoregulatory function.

Control of blood flow

The muscular tone of vessels is controlled by the following factors.

Pressure of the blood within vessels (myogenic theory)

- The myogenic theory was originally described by Bayliss and states that:
  - Increased intraluminal pressure results in constriction of vessels.
  - Decreased intraluminal pressure results in their dilatation.
- This mechanism helps to keep blood flow constant and is the cause of the immediate hyperaemia observed on release of a tourniquet.

Neural innervation

· Arterioles, AVAs and precapillary sphincters are densely innervated by sympathetic fibres.

· Neural control regulates skin blood flow in the following ways.

  · Increased arteriolar tone results in a decrease of cutaneous blood flow.

  · Increased precapillary sphincter tone reduces the blood flow into the capillary networks.

  · Decreased AVA tone results in an increase in the non-nutritive blood flow bypassing the capillary bed.

Humoral factors

· Epinephrine (adrenaline) and norepinephrine (noradrenaline) cause vasoconstriction of the vessels.

· Histamine and bradykinin cause vasodilatation.

· Low oxygen saturation, high carbon dioxide saturation and acidosis also result in vasodilatation.

Temperature

Increased heat produces cutaneous vasodilatation and increased flow which predominantly bypasses the capillary beds via the AVAs.

The delay phenomenon

· Delay is any preoperative manoeuvre that results in increased flap survival.

· Historical examples include Tagliacozzi's technique for nasal reconstruction described in the 16th century.

  · This involves elevation of a bipedicled flap with a length : breadth ratio of 2 : 1 (the flap can be considered as two flaps of the ratio 1 : 1).

  · Cotton lint is then placed under the flap, preventing its reattachment.

  · Two weeks later one end of the flap is detached from the arm and attached to the nose.

  · A flap of these dimensions transferred immediately, without a prior delay procedure, would have an increased chance of distal necrosis.

· A form of delay used in clinical practice today is the division of the DIEA supplying the rectus muscle, 2 weeks prior to pedicled TRAM-flap breast reconstruction.

Despite many advances in our understanding, the mechanism of delay remains incompletely understood. The following theories have been proposed to explain the delay phenomenon.

Increased axiality of blood flow

· Removal of the blood flow from the periphery of a random flap will promote the development of an axial blood supply from its base along its axis.

· Axial flaps are known to have improved survival when compared with random flaps.

Tolerance to ischaemia

- Cells become accustomed to hypoxia after the initial delay procedure.
- Less tissue necrosis therefore occurs after the second operation.

Sympathectomy vasodilatation theory

- Sympathectomy resulting from dividing the sympathetic fibres at the borders of the flap results in vasodilatation and an improved blood supply.
- But why, if sympathectomy is immediate, does the delay phenomenon only begin to appear at 48 h, and why does it take 2 weeks to reach its maximum effect?

Interflap shunting hypothesis

- This theory postulates that sympathectomy dilates the AVAs more than the precapillary sphincters, resulting in an increase in non-nutritive blood flow bypassing the capillary bed.
- A greater length of flap will survive at the second stage as there are fewer sympathetic fibres to cut and therefore there will be less of a reduction in non-nutritive flow.

Hyperadrenergic state

- Surgery results in increased tissue concentrations of vasoconstrictor substances, such as epinephrine and norepinephrine.
- After the initial delay procedure, the resultant reduction in blood supply is not sufficient to produce tissue necrosis.
- The level of vasoconstrictor substances returns to normal before the second procedure.
- The second procedure produces another rise in the concentration of vasoconstrictor substances.
- This rise is smaller than it would be if the flap were elevated without a prior delay.
- The flap is therefore less likely to undergo distal necrosis if a prior delay is performed.

Unifying theory

- This theory was described by Pearl in 1981.
- It incorporates elements of all of the above theories.

Classification of flaps

Flaps can be classified by the five 'C's:

- Circulation
- Composition
- Contiguity
- Contour
- Conditioning.

Circulation

The circulation to flaps can be further subcategorized into:
· Random
· Axial (direct; fasciocutaneous; musculocutaneous; or venous).

Random flaps

· Random flaps have no directional blood supply and are not based on any known vessel.
· These include most local flaps on the face.
· They should have a maximum length : breadth ratio of 1 : 1 in the lower extremity, as it has a poor blood supply.
· They can have a length : breadth ratio of up to 1 : 6 in the face, as it has a good blood supply.

Axial flaps

Direct

· Direct flaps contain a named artery running along the axis of the flap in the subcutaneous tissue.
· Examples include:
  · The groin flap based on the superficial external iliac vessels.
  · The deltopectoral flap based on perforating vessels of the internal mammary artery.
· Both flaps can include a random segment in their distal portions after the artery peters out.

Fasciocutaneous

· Fasciocutaneous flaps are based on vessels running either within or near the fascia.
· Blood reaches these flaps from fasciocutaneous vessels (also called septocutaneous vessels) running from the deep arteries of the body to the fascia.
· The fasciocutaneous system predominates on the limbs and this is the location of most of these flaps.

Fasciocutaneous flaps have been classified by Cormack and Lamberty into the following types:
· *Type A*
  · These flaps are dependent on multiple non-named fasciocutaneous vessels that enter the base of the flap.
  · The lower-leg 'super flaps' described by Pontén are examples of type A flaps. Their dimensions vastly exceed the 1 : 1 ratios recommended for random flaps in the lower leg.
· *Type B*
  · These are based on a single fasciocutaneous vessel which runs along the axis of the flap.
  · Examples include the scapular and parascapular flaps, and the fasciocutaneous flaps based on perforators in the lower leg.

- *Type C*
  - These flaps are supplied by multiple small, perforating vessels which reach the flap from a deep artery running along a fascial septum between muscles.
  - Examples include the radial forearm flap (RFF) and the lateral arm flap.
- *Type D*
  - These are fasciocutaneous flaps that contain bone.
  - As these flaps are usually type C, they have recently been reclassified as 'type C flaps with bone'.
  - Examples include:
    - The RFF raised with a segment of the radius.
    - The lateral arm flap raised with a segment of the lateral supracondylar ridge of the humerus.

Musculocutaneous

- Musculocutaneous flaps are based on perforators that reach the skin through the muscle.
- The musculocutaneous system predominates on the torso and this is the location of most of these flaps.

Musculocutaneous flaps were classified by Mathes and Nahai in 1981.

- *Type 1*
  - These flaps are supplied by a single vascular pedicle.
  - Examples include the gastrocnemius, the tensor fascia lata (TFL) and the abductor digiti minimi (ADM).
  - These are generally good flaps for transfer, as the whole muscle is nourished by a single pedicle.
- *Type 2*
  - These flaps are supplied by a single dominant pedicle which enters the muscle near its origin or insertion point.
  - Additional smaller vascular pedicles enter the muscle belly.
  - Examples include the trapezius, temporalis and gracilis flaps.
  - These are generally good flaps for transfer, as they can be based on the single dominant pedicle.
- *Type 3*
  - These flaps are supplied by two vascular pedicles, each arising from a separate regional artery.
  - Examples include the rectus abdominis and the gluteus maximus flaps.
  - These are useful muscles for transfer, as they can be based on either pedicle.
- *Type 4*
  - These flaps are supplied by multiple segmental pedicles.
  - Examples include the sartorius, the tibialis anterior and the long flexors and extensors of the toes.
  - In practice they are seldom used for transfer, as each pedicle only supplies a small portion of muscle.
- *Type 5*
  - These flaps have one dominant vascular pedicle and secondary smaller segmental pedicles.

  - Examples include the latissimus dorsi and the pectoralis major.
  - These are useful flaps, as they can be based on either the dominant vascular pedicle or the secondary smaller segmental pedicles.

Venous

- These flaps are based on venous rather than arterial pedicles.
- In fact, many of the venous pedicles have very small arteries running alongside them.
- One example is the saphenous flap, which is based on the short saphenous vein and often used to reconstruct defects around the knee.

Venous flaps have been classified by Thatte and Thatte as follows:

- *Type 1*
  - These flaps are supplied by a single venous pedicle.
- *Type 2*
  - These are venous flow-through flaps and are supplied by a vein which enters one side of the flap and exits from the other.
- *Type 3*
  - These are arterialized venous flaps.

Venous flaps tend to become very congested post-operatively and have not been universally accepted.

Composition

Flaps can be classified by their composition, as:

- Cutaneous
- Fasciocutaneous
- Fascial
- Musculocutaneous
- Muscle only
- Osseocutaneous
- Osseous.

Contiguity

Flaps can be classified by their source, as:

- Local flaps
  - These are composed of tissue adjacent to the defect.
- Regional flaps
  - These are composed of tissue from the same region of the body as the defect, e.g. head and neck, upper limb.
- Distant flaps
  - Pedicled distant flaps are from a distant part of the body to which they remain attached.
  - Free flaps are completely detached from the body and anastomosed to recipient vessels close to the defect.

Contour

Flaps can be classified by the method in which they are transferred into the defect. Methods of transferring flaps include the following.

Advancement

The following methods can be used to facilitate advancement of a flap into a defect.

- Stretching of the flap
- Excision of Burow's triangles at its base
- V-Y advancement
- Z-plasty at its base
- A combination of the above.

Transposition

- The flap is moved into a defect from an adjacent position, leaving a defect which must be closed by another method.

Rotation

- The flap is rotated into the defect.
- Classically, rotation flaps are of sufficient dimensions to permit closure of the donor defect.
- In reality, many flaps have elements of transposition and rotation and may be best described as pivot flaps.

Interpolation

- These flaps are moved into a defect either under or above an intervening bridge of tissue.

Crane principle

- This technique aims to transform an ungraftable bed into one that will accept a skin graft.
- At the first stage a flap is placed into the defect.
- After a sufficient time period to allow vascular ingrowth into the flap from the recipient site, the superficial portion of flap is replaced in its original position. This leaves a segment of subcutaneous tissue in the defect, which can now accept a skin graft.

Conditioning

- 'Delay' is any preoperative manoeuvre which will result in increased flap survival.
- Traditionally delay has been used to increase the survival of flaps prior to surgery.
- The mechanism of delay is discussed in more detail in 'The blood supply to the skin' (p. 7).

Geometry of local flaps

Orientation of elective incisions

- In the 19th century, Langer showed that circular awl wounds produced elliptical defects in cadaver skin.
- He believed that this occurred because the skin tension along the longitudinal axis of the ellipse exceeded that along the transverse axis.

- Borges has provided over 36 descriptive terms for skin lines. These include:
  - Relaxed skin tension lines (RSTLs)—these are parallel to the natural skin wrinkles (rhytids) and tend to be perpendicular to the fibres of the underlying muscle.
  - Lines of maximum extensibility (LMEs)—these lie perpendicular to the RSTLs and parallel to the fibres of the underlying muscle.
- The best orientation of an incision can be judged by a number of methods, including:
  - Knowledge of the direction of pull of the underlying muscle.
  - Ascertaining whether the incision is parallel to any rhytids or RSTLs.
  - Ascertaining whether the incision is perpendicular to the LMEs.
  - Ascertaining whether the incision is parallel to the direction of hair growth.
  - 'The pinch test'—if the skin is pinched transversely it will form a transverse fold without distortion if it is orientated correctly; if a sigmoid-shaped fold forms it is orientated incorrectly.

Plasty techniques

Z-plasty

- This technique involves the transposition of two triangular-shaped flaps.
- A Z-plasty can be used to:
  - Increase the length of an area of tissue or a scar
  - Break up a straight-line scar
  - Realign a scar.
- The degree of elongation of the longitudinal axis of the Z-plasty is directly related to the angles of its constituent flaps.

  30° → 25% elongation
  45° → 50% elongation
  60° → 75% elongation
  75° → 100% elongation
  90° → 125% elongation.
- The amount of elongation obtained for each flap angle can be worked out by starting at 30° and 25% and adding 15° and 25% to each of the figures.
- Gains in tissue length are only estimates and depend on local tissue elasticity and tension.
- Flaps of 60° angulation are most commonly used clinically as they provide sufficient lengthening without undue tension.
- The angles of the two flaps do not need to be equal and can be designed to suit local tissue requirements.
- All three limbs should be of the same length.
- The following steps should be taken when designing a Z-plasty to realign a scar.
  1. Mark the desired direction of the scar.
  2. Draw the central limb of the Z-plasty along the original scar.
  3. Draw the lateral limbs of the Z-plasty from the ends of the central limb to a line along the desired direction of the scar.
  4. Two patterns will be available, one with a wide angle at the apex of the flaps, the other with a narrow angle.

5 Select the pattern with the narrower angle as these flaps transpose better than those with a wider angle.

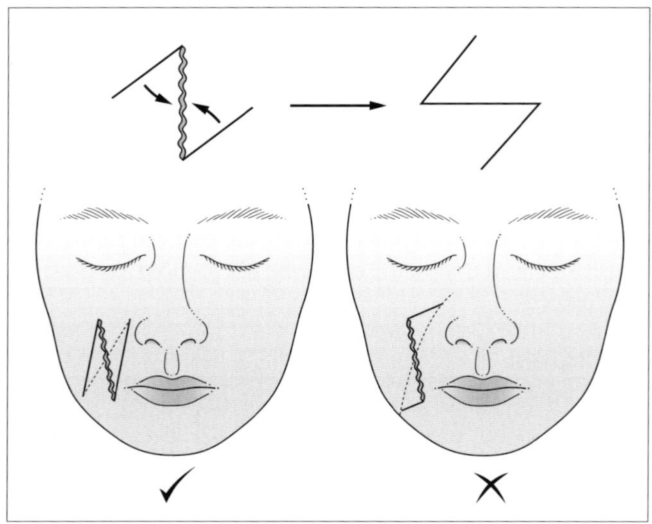

The four-flap plasty

- This technique is used to elongate an area of tissue.
- It is, in effect, two interdependent Z-plasties.
- It can be designed with different angles.
- The two outer flaps become the inner flaps after transposition.
- The two inner flaps become the outer flaps after transposition.
- The flaps, which are originally in an 'ABCD' configuration, end as 'CADB' (**CADB**ury).

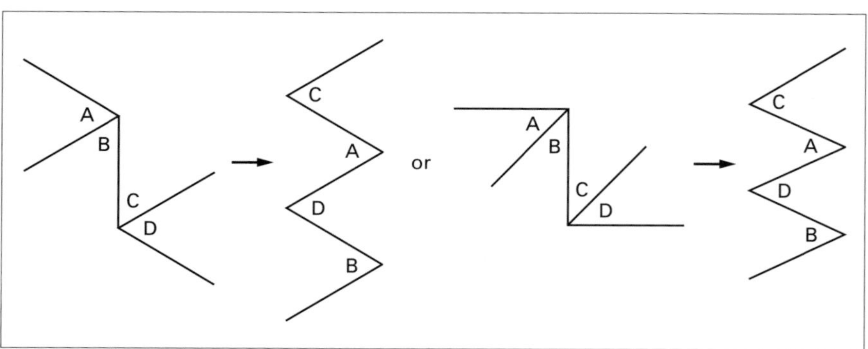

The five-flap plasty

- Because of its appearance this technique is also called a jumping-man flap.
- It is used to elongate tissue and is often utilized clinically to release first web space contractures and epicanthal folds.
- It is, in effect, two opposing Z-plasties with a V-Y advancement in the centre.
- The flaps, which are originally in an 'ABCDE' configuration, end as 'BACED'.

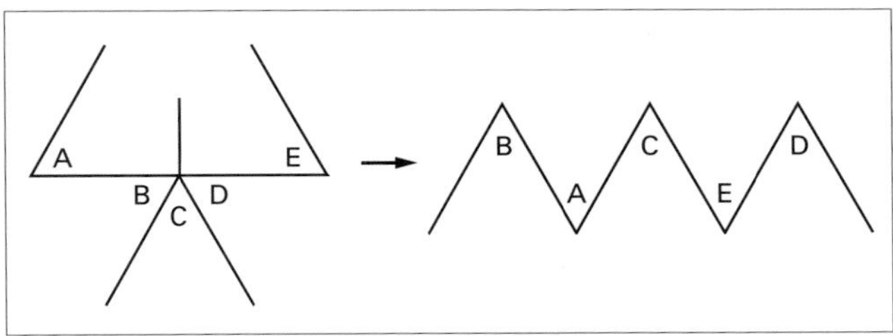

The W-plasty

- This technique is used to break up the line of a scar and improve its aesthetics.
- Unlike the Z-plasty and the four- and five-flap plasties, it does not lengthen tissue.
- If possible, one of the limbs of the W-plasty should lie parallel to the RSTLs so that half of the resultant scar will lie parallel to them.
- This technique involves discarding normal tissue, which may be a disadvantage in certain areas.

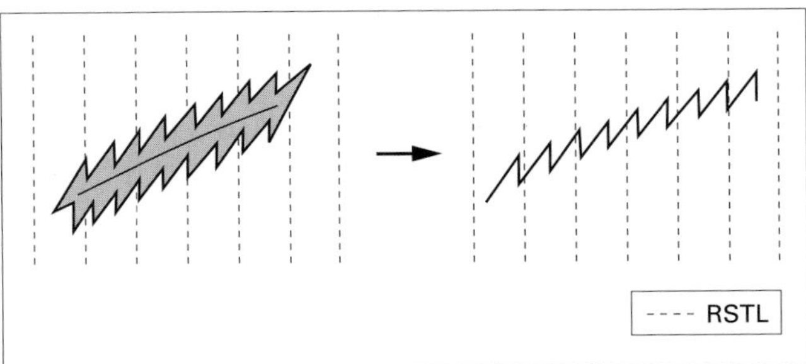

Local flaps

Local flaps may be:

- Advancement flaps (simple; modified; V-Y; or bipedicled).
- Pivot flaps (transposition; interpolation; rotation ; or bilobed).

Advancement flaps

Simple

Simple advancement flaps rely on skin elasticity.

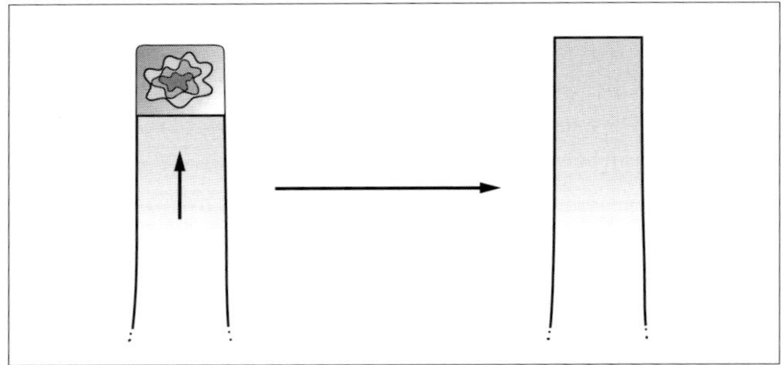

Modified

Modified advancement flaps incorporate one of the following techniques at the base of the flap to increase tissue advancement.

- A counter incision
- A Burow's triangle
- A Z-plasty.

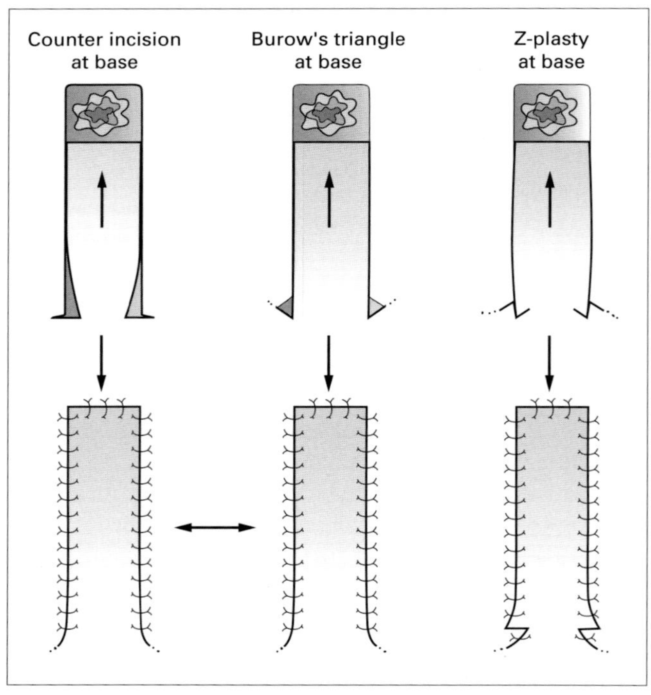

V-Y

· These flaps are incised along each of their cutaneous borders.

· The blood supply to these flaps arises from the deep tissue and passes to the flap through a subcutaneous pedicle.

· Horn flaps and oblique V-Y flaps are modifications of the original V-Y flap.

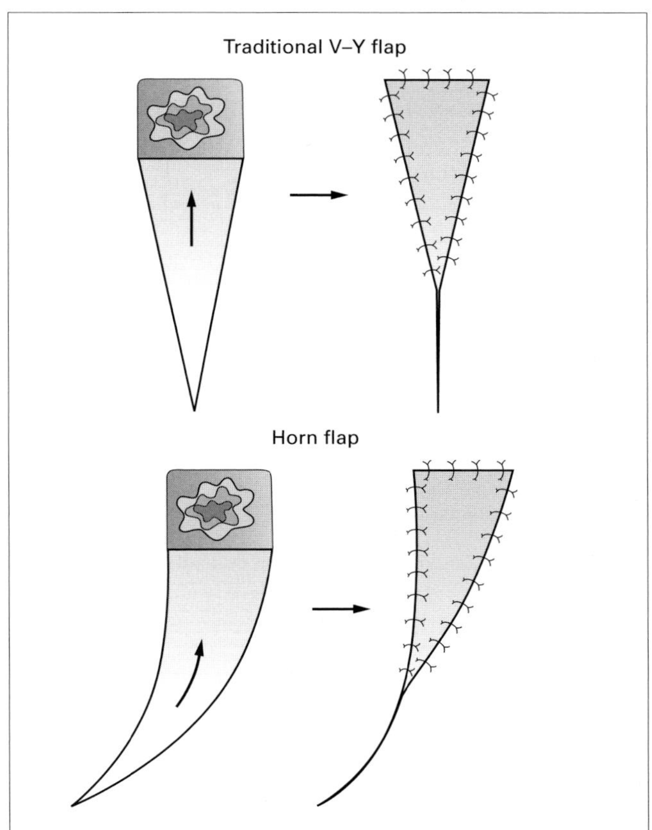

Bipedicled

· These flaps receive a blood supply from both ends.

· They are less prone to necrosis than flaps of similar dimensions, which are only attached at one end.

· A commonly used bipedicled flap is the von Langenbeck mucoperiosteal flap, used to repair cleft palates.

· Bipedicled flaps should be designed with their limbs curved parallel to the circumference of the defect.

· This design permits flap transposition with less tension.

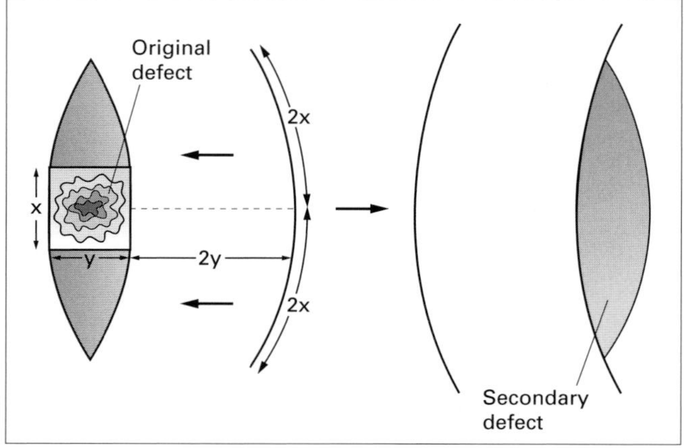

Pivot flaps

Transposition flaps

These flaps are transposed into the defect, leaving a donor site which is closed by some other means (often a skin graft).

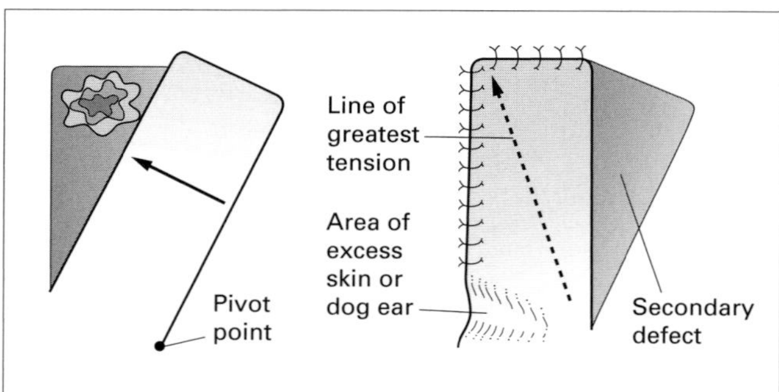

Transposition flaps with direct closure of donor site

- These include the rhomboid flap (Limberg flap) and the Dufourmontel flap.
- These flaps are similar in concept but vary in geometry.
- Both flaps should be designed so as to leave the donor site scar lying parallel to the RSTLs.

The rhomboid flap

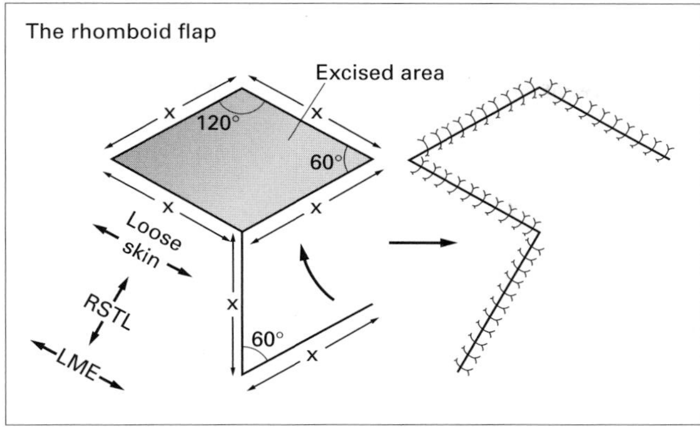

The Dufourmontel flap

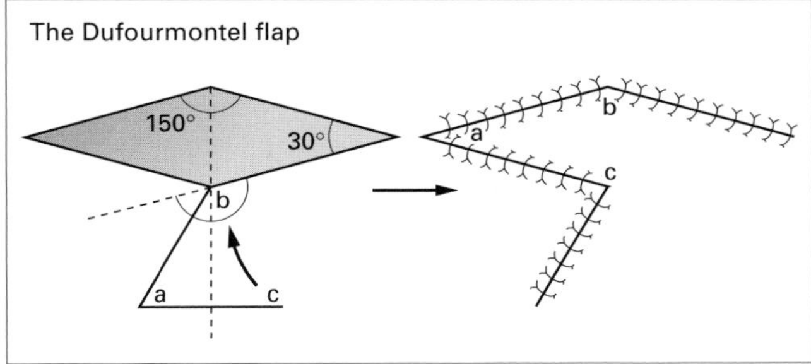

Interpolation flaps

- These flaps are raised from local, but not adjacent, skin.
- The pedicle must therefore be passed either over or under an intervening skin bridge.

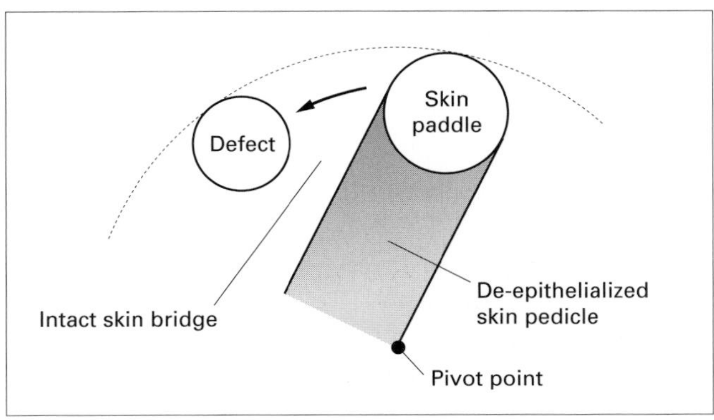

Rotation flaps

- These large flaps rotate tissue into the defect.
- Tissue redistribution usually permits direct closure of the donor site.
- The flap circumference should be 5–8 times the width of the defect.
- Clinically, these flaps are often used on the scalp.
- The back cut at the base of the flap can be directed either towards or away from the defect.

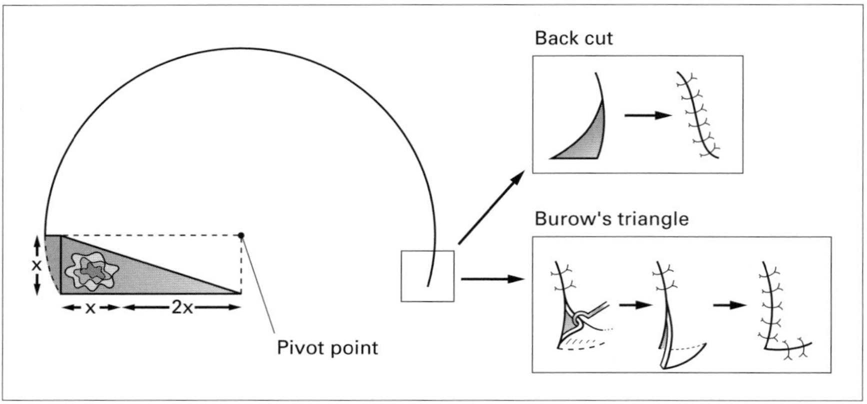

The bilobed flap

- Many varied designs of this flap have been described.
- It consists of two transposition flaps.
- The first flap is transposed into the original defect.
- The second flap is transposed into the secondary defect at the original site of the first flap.
- The tertiary defect at the original site of the second flap should be small enough to close directly.
- The flap should ideally be designed so that this suture line lies parallel to the RSTLs.

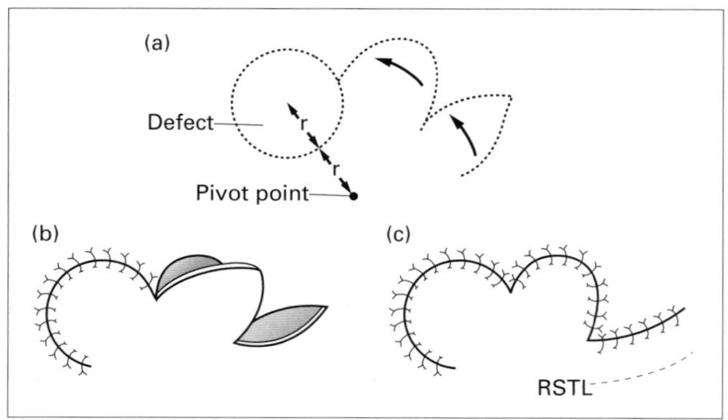

Wound healing and skin grafts

Wound healing can occur by the following methods.

- Healing by primary intention
  - The skin edges are directly opposed.
  - Healing is normally good with minimal scar formation.
- Healing by secondary intention
  - The wound is left open to heal by a combination of contraction and epithelialization.
  - Increased inflammation and proliferation occur in these wounds when compared with those that heal by primary intention.
- Healing by tertiary intention
  - This occurs in wounds that are initially left open, then closed as a secondary procedure.

Phases of wound healing

Wound healing consists of four phases: (i) haemostasis; (ii) inflammation; (iii) proliferation; and (iv) remodelling.

Haemostasis

- The vessels vasoconstrict immediately after division.
- A platelet plug is then formed.
- The platelets degranulate; platelet-derived growth factor (PDGF) and thromboxanes stimulate the conversion of fibrinogen to fibrin. This stimulates propagation of the thrombus.
- The thrombus is initially pale when it contains platelets alone (white thrombus).
- As red blood cells are trapped within it the thrombus becomes darker (red thrombus).

Inflammation

- This phase occurs in the first 2–3 days after injury.
- Its stimulus may be:
  - Physical injury
  - Antigen–antibody reaction
  - Infection.
- The thrombus releases growth factors such as PDGF.
- Endothelial cells swell, allowing the egress of polymorphonuclear lymphocytes (polymorphs or PMNs) and mononuclear cells (monocytes and macrophages) into the surrounding tissue.

Proliferation

- This phase begins on the 2nd or 3rd day following injury and lasts for 2–4 weeks.
- Macrophages within the tissue release growth factors which are chemoattractant to fibroblasts.
- Fibroblasts which are usually located in perivascular tissue migrate along networks of fibrin fibres into the wound.

- The fibroblasts secrete GAGs and produce collagen and elastin.
- GAGs consist of a protein core surrounded by disaccharide units.
- When hydrated, GAGs become ground substance.

Remodelling

- This phase begins 2–4 weeks after injury, as the proliferative phase subsides.
- During the remodelling phase there is no net increase in collagen (state of collagen homeostasis).
- The extensive capillary network produced in the proliferative phase begins to involute.
- The collagen fibres, which are initially laid down in a haphazard manner, become arranged in a more organized manner.

Function of the macrophage in wound healing

- Macrophages are derived from mononuclear leucocytes.
- They debride tissue and remove micro-organisms.
- They co-ordinate the activity of fibroblasts by releasing growth factors.
- These include interleukin 1 (IL-1), tumour necrosis factor alpha (TNF-alpha) and transforming growth factor beta (TGF-beta).
- Macrophages are essential for normal wound healing.
- Wounds depleted of macrophages heal slowly.

Epithelial repair

This process, whereby epithelial continuity is re-established across a wound, consists of the following four phases.

Mobilization

1 Epithelial cells at the wound edges enlarge and flatten.
2 They detach from the neighbouring cells and the basement membrane.
3 They then move away from adjoining cells.

Migration

1 Decreased contact inhibition promotes cell migration.
2 The cells migrate across the wound until they meet those from the opposite wound edge.
3 At this point, contact inhibition is reinstituted and migration ceases.

Mitosis

Epithelial cells begin to proliferate once they have covered the surface of the wound.

Cellular differentiation

1 The normal structure of stratified squamous epithelium is re-established.
2 The cells differentiate and the layered structure of stratified squamous epithelium is reconstituted.

Collagen

- Collagen constitutes approximately 30% of the total body protein.
- Collagen is formed by the hydroxylation of the aminoacids lysine and proline.
- Procollagen is initially formed within the cell.
- Procollagen is transformed into tropocollagen after it is excreted from the cell.
- Fully formed collagen has a complex structure.
  - It consists of three polypeptide chains wound in a left-handed helix.
  - These three chains are further wound in a right-handed coil to form the basic tropocollagen unit.
- Collagen formation is inhibited by colchicine, penicillamide, steroids, vitamin C and iron deficiency.
- There are at least five types of collagen. Each type of collagen shares the same basic structure but differs in the relative composition of hydroxylysine and hydroxyproline and in the degree of cross-linking between chains.
  - *Type 1*: predominant in mature skin, bone and tendon.
  - *Type 2*: present in hyaline cartilage and the cornea.
  - *Type 3*: present in healing tissue, particularly in fetal wounds.
  - *Type 4*: predominant constituent of basement membranes.
  - *Type 5*: similar to type 4 and also found in the basement membrane.
- The ratio of type 1 collagen : type 3 collagen in normal skin is 5 : 1.
- Hypertrophic and immature scars contain a ratio of 2 : 1 or less.
- 90% of the total body collagen is type 1.

The myofibroblast

- This cell was first identified by Gabbiani in 1971.
- It resembles a fibroblast but differs in that it contains cytoplasmic filaments of α-smooth muscle actin.
- α-smooth muscle actin is also found in smooth muscle.
- The muscle fibres within the fibroblast are thought to be responsible for wound contraction.
- The number of myofibroblasts within a wound is proportional to its contraction.
- Increased numbers of myofibroblasts have been found in the fascia in patients with Dupuytren's disease.
- They are thought to be responsible for the abnormal contraction of this tissue.

TGF-β

- This growth factor is secreted by macrophages. It is believed to play a central role in wound healing and has a number of effects including:
  - Chemoattraction of fibroblasts and macrophages
  - Induction of angiogenesis
  - Stimulation of extracellular matrix deposition.
- Three isoforms of TGF-β have been identified.
  - Types 1 and 2 promote wound healing and scarring.
  - Type 3 decreases wound healing and scarring and in the future may have a role as an antiscarring agent.

· TGF-β is not present in fetal wounds and this may be one of the factors responsible for the decreased inflammation and improved scarring observed in this tissue.

Factors affecting healing

Factors affecting wound healing may be: (i) systemic (congenital or acquired); or (ii) local.

Systemic factors: congenital

Pseudoxanthoma elasticum

- This is an autosomal recessive condition.
- It is characterized by increased collagen degradation.
- The skin is pebbled and extremely lax.

Ehlers–Danlos syndrome

- This is a heterogeneous collection of connective tissue disorders.
- It results from defects in the synthesis, structure or cross-linking of collagen.
- Clinical features include:
  - Hypermobile fingers
  - Hyperextensible skin
  - Fragile connective tissues.
- Surgery should be avoided if possible in these patients as wound healing is poor.

Cutis laxa

- This condition presents in the neonatal period.
- The skin is abnormally lax.
- Typically the patient has coarsely textured, drooping skin.

Progeria

- This condition is characterized by premature ageing.
- Clinical features of the condition include:
  - Growth retardation
  - Baldness
  - Atherosclerosis.

Werner syndrome

- This is an autosomal recessive condition.
- Skin changes are similar to scleroderma.
- Elective surgery should be avoided whenever possible as healing is poor.

Epidermolysis bullosa

- This is a heterogeneous collection of separate conditions.
- The skin is very susceptible to mechanical stress.
- Blistering may occur after minor trauma (Nikolsky sign).

· The most severe subtype, dermolytic bullous dermatitis (DBD), results in hand fibrosis and syndactyly.

Systemic factors: acquired

Nutrition

· Vitamin A deficiency delays wound healing.
· Vitamin C is required for collagen synthesis.
· Vitamin E acts as a membrane stabilizer; deficiency may inhibit healing.
· Zinc is a constituent of many enzymes; administration accelerates healing in deficient states.
· Albumin is an indicator of malnutrition; low levels are associated with poor healing.

Pharmacological

· Steroids decrease inflammation and subsequent wound healing.
· Non-steroidal anti-inflammatory drugs (NSAIDs) decrease collagen synthesis.

Endocrine abnormalities

· Diabetics often have delayed wound healing.
· Recent evidence suggests neuropathy rather than small vessel occlusive disease may be responsible for the delayed healing (see 'Leg ulcers', p. 244).

Age

· The rate of cell multiplication decreases with age.
· All stages of wound healing are more protracted in the elderly.
· Healed wounds have decreased tensile strength in the elderly.

Smoking

· Nicotine is a sympathetic stimulant which causes vasoconstriction and consequently decreases tissue perfusion.
· Carbon dioxide, contained in cigarette smoke, shifts the oxygen dissociation curve and reduces tissue oxygenation.

Local factors

Infection

· Subclinical wound infection can impair wound healing.
· Wounds with over 10^5 organisms per gram of tissue are considered infected and are unlikely to heal without further treatment.

Radiation

· Radiation causes endothelial cell, capillary and arteriole damage.
· Irradiated fibroblasts secrete less collagen and extracellular matrix.
· Lymphatics are also damaged, resulting in oedema and an increased risk of infection.

Blood supply

- Decreased tissue perfusion results in decreased wound oxygenation.
- Fibroblasts are oxygen-sensitive and their function is reduced in hypoxic tissue.
- Reduced oxygen delivery to the tissues can result from decreases in:
  - Inspired oxygen concentration
  - Oxygen transfer to haemoglobin
  - Haemoglobin concentration
  - Tissue perfusion.
- Decreased oxygen delivery to the tissue reduces:
  - Collagen formation
  - Extracellular matrix deposition
  - Angiogenesis
  - Epithelialization.
- Hyperbaric oxygen treatment increases the inspired oxygen concentration but its effectiveness relies on good tissue perfusion.

Trauma

The delicate neoepidermis of healing wounds is disrupted by trauma.

Neural supply

- There is some evidence that wounds in denervated tissue heal slowly.
- This may contribute to the delayed wound healing observed in some pressure sores, and in patients with diabetes and leprosy.

Fetal wound healing

- Tissue healing during the first 3 months of fetal life occurs by regeneration rather than by scarring.
- Regenerative healing is characterized by the absence of scarring.
- Regenerative wound healing differs from normal adult healing in the following ways.
  - Inflammation is reduced.
  - Epithelialization is more rapid.
  - Angiogenesis is reduced.
  - Collagen deposition is rapid, not excessive and organized.
  - More type 3 rather than type 1 collagen is laid down.
  - The wound contains a greater proportion of water and hyaluronic acid.
- The lack of TGF-β in fetal wounds may be responsible for some of these differences.

Skin grafts

- Skin grafts are either full or split thickness.
- Split-skin grafts contain a variable amount of dermis and are usually harvested from the thigh or buttock.
- Full-thickness skin grafts contain the entire dermis and are usually harvested from areas with sufficient tissue laxity to permit direct closure of the donor defect.

- Primary contraction is the immediate recoil observed in freshly harvested skin.
- Secondary contraction occurs after the graft is applied to its bed.
- The thinner the graft, the greater the degree of secondary contraction.

Mechanisms

Skin grafts heal in four phases.

Adherence

- Fibrin bonds form immediately on applying a skin graft to a suitable recipient bed.

Serum imbibition

- Skin grafts swell in the first 2–4 days after application.
- This increase in volume results from absorption of fluid (serum imbibition).
- The nutritive value of serum imbibition in maintaining graft viability is debated.

Revascularization

- Vessel ingrowth into skin grafts begins on about the 4th day.
- The mechanism of revascularization is uncertain and may be via:
  - Inosculation—direct anastomosis between the vessels within the graft and those in the recipient tissue.
  - Revascularization—new vessel ingrowth from the recipient tissue along the vascular channels of the graft.
  - Neovascularization—new vessel ingrowth from the recipient tissue along new channels in the graft.

Remodelling

This is the process whereby the histological architecture of the graft returns to that of normal skin.

Reasons for graft failure

Skin grafts fail for the following reasons.

Haematoma

- This is the most common cause of graft failure.
- The risk of haematoma formation is minimized by:
  - Meticulous haemostasis
  - The use of a meshed skin graft which allows blood to escape
  - The application of a pressure dressing.

Infection

- Generally, skin grafts will not take if the bacterial count of the donor site exceeds 10^5 organisms per gram.
- Some organisms such as the beta haemolytic streptococcus can destroy grafts when present in much fewer numbers.

Seroma
Any collection of fluid under the graft reduces the likelihood of its taking successfully.

Shear
- This is a lateral force placed on a graft.
- It results in the disruption of the delicate connections between the graft and its bed and consequently reduces the likelihood of successful graft take.

Inappropriate bed
- Skin grafts will not survive on cartilage, tendon and endochondral bone denuded of periosteum.
- Membranous bone, found in some areas of the skull, will accept a skin graft.
- Grafts on previously irradiated tissue are prone to failure.

Technical error
- An assortment of technical errors can result in graft failure.
- Examples include placing the graft upside down or allowing it to dry out before application.

Bone healing and bone grafts

- All bones are derived from mesenchyme.
- All are composed of an organic matrix (osteoid) which is mineralized by the calcium salt hydroxyapatite.

Bones are formed by one of two different mechanisms: (i) intramembranous ossification; or (ii) endochondral ossification.

Intramembranous ossification
- Bones formed by intramembranous ossification include the flat bones of the face, calvarium and ribs.
- Intramembranous ossification occurs by direct deposition of bone within a vascularized membranous template.

Endochondral ossification
- Endochondral bones develop from a cartilage precursor.
- Bones formed by endochondral ossification include all the long bones and the iliac crest.

Bone structure

- All bones have an outer cortical layer and an inner cancellous layer.
- The cancellous portion of membranous bone is found within the diploic space.
- Cancellous bone consists of loosely woven trabeculae made up of organic and inorganic bone.

- Cortical bone consists of:
  - Multiple bone units (osteons), which are composed of a central longitudinal canal (haversian canal) that contains a central blood vessel.
  - The osteons are interconnected by transverse nutrient canals (Volkmann canals).
  - Bone is laid down in concentric layers around each haversian canal.
  - Osteocytes are scattered throughout the osteons.

Blood supply to bone

Blood reaches bone by one of the following routes:

1 Periosteal vessels at the sites of muscle attachments
2 Apophyseal vessels at the sites of tendon and ligament attachment
3 Nutrient arteries supplying the medullary cavity
4 Epiphyseal vessels supplying the growth plates.

Bone healing

The phases of bone healing are similar to those of wound healing.

1 Haematoma formation
2 Inflammation
3 Cellular proliferation
   - Periosteal proliferation occurs on the outer aspect of the cortex.
   - Endosteal proliferation occurs on the inner aspect of the cortex.
4 Callus formation
   - Callus consists of immature woven bone composed of osteoid laid down by osteoblasts.
   - This osteoid is mineralized with hydroxyapatite.
5 Remodelling
   - The cortical structure and medullary cavity are restored.

Primary healing

- This occurs if bone is rigidly fixed with direct apposition of the bone ends.
- Primary bone healing is characterized by restoration of the normal bone structure.
- The inflammatory and proliferative phases of bone healing do not occur.
- Callus is not formed.

Secondary healing

- This occurs if the fragments are not rigidly fixed, or if a gap exists between the bone ends.

Complications of fractures

These include:

- Delayed union
- Non-union
- Mal-union
- Infection

- Avascular necrosis (AVN)
- Shortening
- Damage to adjacent structures.

Bone graft healing

Bone grafts heal by the following mechanisms.

Incorporation

- This is adherence of the graft to the host tissue.
- Incorporation is maximized in immobilized, well-vascularized tissue.

Osseoconduction

- The bone graft acts as a scaffold along which vessels and osteoprogenitor cells travel.
- Old bone is absorbed as new is deposited.
- This process is also known as creeping substitution.

Osseoinduction

- This is the differentiation of mesenchymal cells within the local tissue into osteocytes.
- Osteoclasts, osteoblasts and osteocytes within the bone graft are not capable of mitosis.
- The increased numbers of these cells within the bone graft are derived from the mesenchymal tissue of the recipient site.
- Osseoinduction is controlled by bone morphogenic proteins (BMPs).

Osteogenesis

- This is the formation of new bone by surviving cells within the bone graft.
- It is the predominant mechanism by which new bone is formed in vascularized bone grafts.
- Osteogenesis does not occur to a significant degree in non-vascularized bone grafts.

Survival of bone grafts

Factors influencing the survival of bone grafts can be divided into three groups: (i) systemic factors; (ii) intrinsic graft factors; and (iii) factors relating to the placement of the graft.

Systemic factors

These are similar to those affecting wound healing and include:

- Age
- Nutrition
- Immunosuppression
- Drugs
- Diabetes
- Obesity.

Intrinsic graft factors

· Bone grafts with intact periosteum undergo less absorption than those stripped of this covering.
· Membranous bone undergoes less absorption than endochondral bone when used as an onlay graft in the facial skeleton.

Graft placement factors

Orthotopic or heterotopic placement

· Orthotopic—graft is placed into a position normally occupied by bone.
· Heterotopic—graft is placed into a position not normally occupied by bone.
· Grafts placed into an orthotopic position are less prone to absorption.

Quality of the recipient bed

· Radiotherapy, scarring and infection adversely affect graft survival.

Graft fixation

· Rigidly fixed grafts survive better than those that are mobile.

Site of graft placement

· Grafts survive better in areas in which bone is normally laid down (depository sites).
· These sites include areas such as the zygoma and mandible in the child.

Nerve healing and nerve grafts

Nerve anatomy and function

· Nerve cells (neurons) consist of a cell body from which nerve fibres project.
· Efferent nerve fibres are called axons.
· Afferent nerve fibres are called dendrites.
· The endoneurium surrounds individual nerve fibres or axons.
· The perineurium surrounds groups of nerve fibres (fascicles).
· The epineurium surrounds a group of fascicles to form a peripheral somatic nerve.
· Schwann cells produce a multilaminated myelin sheath in myelinated nerves.
· Unmyelinated nerves are surrounded by a double layer of basement membrane.
· In myelinated nerves, adjacent Schwann cells abut at the nodes of Ranvier.
· Nerve conduction involves the passage of an action potential along a nerve.
· In myelinated nerves, this is via saltatory conduction between adjacent nodes of Ranvier.

Nerve fibres are subdivided into the following groups.

· *Group A*
  · Group A-alpha fibres conduct motor and proprioceptive impulses.
  · Group A-beta fibres transmit pressure and proprioceptive impulses.
  · Group A-gamma fibres conduct motor impulses to the muscle spindles.
  · Group A-delta fibres transmit touch, pain and temperature impulses.

- *Group B*
  - These fibres are found in myelinated, preganglionic autonomic nerves.
- *Group C*
  - These fibres are found in myelinated, postganglionic autonomic nerves.

Medical Research Council grading of nerve function

The MRC have recommended the following grading of nerve function.

Motor function		Sensory function	
M0	No contraction	S0	No sensation
M1	Flicker	S1	Pain sensation
M2	Movement with gravity eliminated	S2	Pain and some touch sensation, possible hypersensitivity
M3	Movement against gravity	S3	Pain and touch with over-reaction
M4	Movement against gravity and resistance	S3+	Some 2-point discrimination
M5	Normal	S4	Normal

Injury

- After transection of a nerve, traumatic degeneration occurs proximally as far as the last node of Ranvier.
- Distally, nerves undergo wallerian degeneration.
- This process was described by Waller in 1850 and consists of:
  - Degeneration of axons and myelin which are then phagocytosed by macrophages and Schwann cells.
  - Collapsed columns of nerve cells develop a bandlike appearance on electron microscopy; these are known as the bands of Buengner.
- Neurotropism is selective, directional growth of nerve fibres towards their appropriate receptors.
- It is mediated by nerve growth factors and consists of the following stages.
  1. The proximal nerve stump sprouts many new fibres.
  2. Fibres growing in an inappropriate direction atrophy.
  3. Those growing in the correct direction survive and grow.
- Neurotropism is non-selective, non-directional growth of nerve fibres.
- Factors which mediate neurotropism include growth factors, extracellular matrix components and hormones.

Classification of nerve injury

- The degree of nerve injury has been classified by both Seddon and Sunderland.
- Seddon classified nerve damage into three groups:
  1. Neurapraxia
  2. Axonotmesis
  3. Neurotmesis.
- Sunderland expanded this classification to five groups.

- **First-degree injury**
  - The axon remains in continuity although conduction is impaired.
  - Recovery should be complete.
- **Second-degree injury**
  - Axonal injury occurs and the segment of nerve distal to the site of damage undergoes wallerian degeneration.
  - All connective tissue layers remain intact and recovery should be good.
- **Third-degree injury**
  - The axon and endoneurium are divided.
  - The perineurium and epineurium remain intact.
  - Recovery should be reasonable.
- **Fourth-degree injury**
  - Complete division of all intraneural structures occurs.
  - The epineurium remains intact.
  - Recovery of some function is expected.
  - This injury may result in neuroma-in-continuity.
- **Fifth-degree injury**
  - The nerve trunk is completely divided.

A sixth-degree injury is added by some to the classification, although it was not described by Sunderland.

- This stage consists of a mixed pattern of nerve injury with segmental damage.
- Seddon's classification of neurapraxia equates to a Sunderland first-degree injury.
- Axonotmesis equates to a second-, third- or fourth-degree injury.
- Neurotmesis equates to a fifth-degree injury.

Nerve repair

- Nerve repair should be performed by direct approximation of the divided stumps whenever possible.
- The ends of the nerve should be trimmed and an epineural repair performed with fine sutures, under magnification.
- Attempts should be made to correctly align the fascicles of the nerve trunks.
- The repair should not be under undue tension.
- Some authorities maintain that primary repair should only be performed in cases in which a single 8/0 suture is strong enough to oppose the divided nerve ends.

Fascicular identification

The following methods can be used to aid fascicular matching during nerve repair.

Matching of anatomical structures during repair

Anatomical guides to the correct orientation of the nerve stumps include:

- The size and orientation of the fascicles
- The distribution of the vessels on the surface of the nerve.

Electrical stimulation

- Motor nerves respond to electrical stimulation for approximately 72 h following division.
- Electrical stimulation of the distal nerve stump during this period can be used to differentiate motor from sensory fibres.
- Awake stimulation of the nerves can be used to differentiate motor from sensory fibres in the proximal nerve stump.
- Electrical stimulation of sensory fibres produces sharp pain.
- Similar stimulation of motor fibres is felt as a dull ache.

Knowledge of internal nerve topography

- The fascicular layout of many nerves is known and can be used to aid accurate repair.
- Ulnar-nerve motor fascicles lie centrally between the volar sensory branches coming from the palm and the dorsal sensory branches coming from the dorsum of the hand.

Nerve grafts

- Nerve grafts are required if primary nerve repair is not possible without undue tension.
- If the divided nerve is large, multiple cables of a smaller donor nerve may be required to bridge the defect.
- It may be possible to reduce the tension across the repair by mobilizing the nerve stumps proximally or distally.
- Methods by which extra nerve length can be obtained by proximal dissection include:
  - Transposition of the ulnar nerve at the elbow.
  - Intratemporal dissection of the facial nerve.
- Materials used to bridge nerve gaps are either autologous or synthetic.
- Of these, autologous nerve is the best material for bridging nerve gaps at present.

Composition

- Autologous tissues that can be used as nerve grafts include:
  - Fresh nerve
  - Freeze–thawed muscle
  - Segments of vein.
- Synthetic nerve grafts composed of fibronectin mats impregnated with growth factors may be available in the future.

Autologous grafts

The following nerves can be used as autologous grafts.

Sural nerve

- This nerve passes behind the lateral malleolus.
- Proximally it divides into the medial sural nerve and the peroneal communicating branch.

- Graft lengths of up to 30–40 cm are available in the adult.
- Endoscopic harvesting has been reported; this produces less scarring.

Lateral antebrachial cutaneous nerve

- This nerve lies adjacent to the cephalic vein alongside the ulnar border of the brachioradialis.
- Graft lengths of up to 8 cm in length are available.
- Removal of this nerve results in only a limited loss of sensation due to cutaneous sensory overlap.

Medial antebrachial cutaneous nerve

- This is located in the groove between triceps and biceps, alongside the basilic vein.
- Distally, it divides into anterior and posterior branches.
- Graft lengths of up to 20 cm are available.

The terminal branch of the posterior interosseous nerve

- This nerve is useful for bridging small defects in small diameter nerves.
- It is located in the radial side of the base of the fourth extensor compartment at the wrist.
- Only a relatively short length of nerve graft is available.

Principles

The following principles are universal to all nerve grafts.

- Both nerve ends should be trimmed back to healthy tissue.
- The graft should be placed in a healthy vascular bed.
- Tension on the graft should be avoided.
- The level of repair should be staggered between the separate cables.
- Wherever possible, the cables should be separated from one another as they bridge the defect.

Tendon healing

Anatomy

- Tendons are composed of dense, metabolically-active connective tissue.
- Within their substance, collagen bundles are arranged in a regular spiraling fashion.
- The collagen is predominantly type 3 with a small amount of type 1.
- Tendons contain few cells; those that are present include:
  - Tenocytes
  - Synovial cells
  - Fibroblasts.
- Endotendon surrounds tendons whilst they lie within synovial sheaths.
- Paratendon is a loose adventitial layer that surrounds tendons outside synovial sheaths.

- Verdan described five zones of flexor tendon injury.
  - *Zone 1*: distal to the insertion of flexor digitorum superficialis (FDS).
  - *Zone 2*: between the proximal end of the flexor sheath and the insertion of FDS.
  - *Zone 3*: between the distal edge of the flexor retinaculum and the proximal end of the flexor sheath.
  - *Zone 4*: under the flexor retinaculum.
  - *Zone 5*: proximal to the flexor retinaculum.
- Zone 2 was described as 'no man's land' by Bunnell because of the poor results of flexor tendon repair at this site.
- Tendon repair in this area is complicated by the fact that the superficial and deep flexors are in close approximation within a tight sheath.
- Extensor tendons are subdivided into eight zones.
  - *Zone 1*: over the distal interphalangeal joint (DIPJ).
  - *Zone 2*: between the proximal interphalangeal joint (PIPJ) and the DIPJ.
  - *Zone 3*: over the PIPJ.
  - *Zone 4*: between the metacarpophalangeal joint (MCPJ) and the PIPJ.
  - *Zone 5*: over the MCPJ.
  - *Zone 6*: between the MCPJ and the extensor retinaculum.
  - *Zone 7*: under the extensor retinaculum.
  - *Zone 8*: between the extensor retinaculum and the musculotendinous junction.
- The odd-numbered zones are located over the joints.
- The first five zones are in the finger.

Mechanisms of tendon healing

Extrinsic healing

- Extrinsinc healing is dependent on fibrous attachments forming between the tendon sheath and the underlying tendon.
- Historically this was believed to be the sole mechanism by which tendons healed.
- This led to the development of post-operative protocols which immobilized the tendons in the mistaken belief that this maximized tendon repair.

Intrinsic healing

- Intrinsic tendon healing is dependent on:
  - Bloodflow though the long and short vinculae.
  - Diffusion from the synovial fluid.
- Lunborg showed that tendons heal when wrapped in a semipermeable membrane and placed in the knee joint of a rabbit.
- Enclosing the tendons in semipermeable membrane stimulates intrinsic healing as it permits the passage of nutrients but not cells.
- Awareness of the ability of tendons to heal by intrinsic mechanisms has led to the development of post-operative protocols which include early mobilization.

Phases of tendon healing

These are similar to those of wound healing.

Inflammation

- This occurs in the first 2–3 days following tendon injury.
- Inflammatory cells infiltrate the wound.
- These cells secrete growth factors which attract fibroblasts.

Proliferation

- This starts 2–3 days after tendon injury and lasts approximately 3 weeks.
- Fibroblasts are responsible for tissue proliferation.
- They manufacture and secrete collagen and GAGs.
- Collagen is initially arranged randomly, consequently the tendon lacks tensile strength.

Remodelling

- This begins approximately 3 weeks following tendon injury.
- It is characterized by collagen homeostasis (the net amount of collagen in the wound remains stable).
- The structure of the tendon differentiates into an organized structure.
- Early motion of the tendon limits the formation of fibrous attachments between itself and the tendon sheath.
- Early motion promotes intrinsic healing at the expense of extrinsic healing.
- Mobilized tendons are stronger than immobilized tendons.

Techniques of repair

Many methods of tendon repair have been described. The following principles apply to most techniques.

- The number and size of the incisions in the flexor sheath should be minimized.
- The A2 and A4 pulleys should be preserved wherever possible.
- Any incision in the sheath should be made between the annular pulleys.
- The tendon ends should be touched as little as possible to protect their delicate covering and reduce the risk of adhesion formation.
- The epitendinous suture in the posterior wall is usually performed first to correctly align the tendon.
- This suture should be inverting and is generally continuous.
- Many designs of core suture have been described, amongst the more commonly used are the:
  - Bunnell stitch
  - Kessler stitch
  - Modified Kessler stitch.
- These suture patterns are usually self locking.
- Two or four strands of core suture are usually used to bridge the gap between the tendons.
- The tendon sheath should be reconstructed when possible but may be left unrepaired in part, if it involves compromising tendon glide.
- In tendon grafts and transfers, the extra length of available tendon allows the ends to be woven into each other, rather than be repaired end-to-end.

- Tendon weaves are more secure than end-to-end repairs.
- The technique most commonly used was described by Pulvertaft and is known as the Pulvertaft weave.
- In this technique the tendons are woven together by passing their ends through three or four longitudinal slits in the body of the other tendon.

Rehabilitation following repair of flexor tendons

- Until relatively recently, tendons were immobilized post-operatively.
- There is now a trend towards earlier mobilization.

The post-operative rehabilitation regimens may consist of the following.

Immobilization

Immobilization is used mainly in children and adults considered unsuitable for early mobilization.

Early passive mobilization

- This involves regular passive motion of the joints.
- No active movement is permitted.

Early active extension with passive flexion

- This regimen was advocated by Kleinert *et al.*
- A dorsal splint protects against hyperextension.
- Finger flexion is maintained by rubber-band traction.
- The rubber bands are attached to the fingernail and the volar aspect of the splint.
- Active extension can occur against the elastic recoil of the bands.
- Passive flexion occurs by the elastic recoil of the bands.

Early active mobilization

- The 'Belfast' regimen is widely used.
- This involves the fitting of a dorsal splint which leaves the fingers free to flex.
- The splint should hold the wrist between neutral and 30° of flexion.
- It should limit MCP extension to 70° of flexion.
- It should limit hyperextension of the interphalangeal joints (IPJs) beyond the neutral position.
- The fingers are left free on their volar surfaces.
- Active mobilization is started in the early post-operative period. This consists of the following three elements.

Passive flexion

This mobilizes the joints and prevents their contraction.

Passive flexion and hold

- This produces an isometric force on the proximal muscle bellies.
- This helps to maintain their function.

Active flexion

- This results in tendon glide within the flexor sheath.
- It limits the formation of fibrous attachments and increases the rate of intrinsic healing.
- The strength of the tendon repair is increased by early active flexion.

Transplantation

- Transplantation is the movement of tissue from one body location to another.
- Orthotopic transfers are transplants into an anatomically similar site.
- Heterotopic transfers are transplants into an anatomically different site.

The following types of transplantation are available.

Autografts

- This is transplantation of tissue from one location to another within the same individual.
- It includes all flaps and grafts.
- Flaps carry with them some intrinsic blood supply; grafts do not.

Isografts

This is transplantation of tissue between genetically identical individuals.

Allografts

- These are also called homografts.
- This is transplantation between different individuals of the same species.

Xenografts

- These were previously called heterografts.
- This is transplantation between individuals of differing species.

Transplant immunology

History

- Gibson and Medawar did much of the pioneering work on transplant immunology in the 1940s and 1950s.
- They described the second set phenomenon, which they defined as 'the accelerated rejection of allogenic tissue due to the presence of humoral antibodies from prior exposure to the same allogenic source'.
- The first set reaction occurs when a skin allograft is applied to an individual for the first time.
- The first set reaction is characterized by the following stages.

1. During the first 1–3 days, allografts behave in a similar fashion to autografts in that they develop dilated capillaries with no blood flow.
2. Between 4 and 7 days, the grafts are infiltrated by leucocytes and thrombi, and punctate haemorrhages appear within their vessels.

3 Between 7 and 8 days, blood flow ceases and the skin graft undergoes necrosis.

- The second set reaction occurs in patients who have been previously grafted with the same allograft material.
- The second set reaction is characterized by the following stages.

1 Immediate hyperacute rejection.

2 The graft never undergoes any revascularization and has been termed a 'white graft'.

Immunology

- Rejection occurs when the host immune system recognizes foreign antigens.
- Foreign antigens are from the major histocompatibility complex (MHC).
- In humans these are known as human leucocyte antigens (HLAs).
- HLAs are six closely linked genes on the short arm of chromosome 6 and are divided into two classes.
  - *Class 1*: includes HLAs A, B and C which are found on all nucleated cells and platelets.
  - *Class 2*: includes HLAs DR, DQ and DP which are found on monocytes, macrophages and both B and T lymphocytes.
- HLAs, A, B and DR are the most important mediators of tissue rejection.

Antigen-presenting cells (APCs), such as macrophages, pick up HLAs from allograft tissue and present them to the host immune system.

- APCs can be of:
  - Donor origin (known as direct presentation)
  - Host origin (known as indirect presentation).
- The host immune system reacts by:
  - Increasing production of IL-1 and IL-2.
  - This causes a rapid clonal expansion in the numbers of T and B lymphocytes within lymphoid tissue.

Graft destruction is produced in the following ways:

1 Direct destruction

- This is mediated by the cellular system.
- CD4 and CD8 cytotoxic T cells cause damage to the graft.

2 Indirect destruction

- This is mediated by the humoral system.
- Stimulated B lymphocytes produce an antibody that binds with the antigen and stimulates tissue destruction via the complement system.

Xenografts

- In transplants between species, natural antibodies often exist without prior sensitization.
- If natural antibodies are present, hyperacute rejection results, occurs secondary to complement activation.
- Concordant transplantation occurs when natural antibodies between species are not present, e.g. primate to human.

· Discordant transplantation occurs when natural antibodies are present, e.g. pig to human.

Immunosuppression

Immunosuppressive techniques can be subdivided into non-specific and specific modalities. Non-specific techniques of immunosuppression include the following.

Radiation

- Whole-body radiation removes mature lymphocytes.
- This technique is not used in humans.
- Localized lymphoid-tissue irradiation is more specifically targeted.
- Graft irradiation aims to try and reduce its antigenicity.

Drugs

- Steroids have an anti-inflammatory and immunosuppressive action.
- Azathioprine downgrades the lymphocyte-activation cascade.
- Cyclosporin is a fungus derivative, isolated in 1976.
- Cyclosporin inhibits the production of IL-2.

Biological agents

- Anti-lymphocyte serum is made by injecting another species with lymphoid tissue from the recipient.
- The anti-lymphocyte antigens produced are powerful suppressers of T-cell activity.

One specific technique of immunosupression is the administration of monoclonal anti-T-lymphocyte antibodies. In the future, monoclonal antibodies may be available to down-regulate specific parts of the immune response.

Alloplastic implantation

The ideal implant should be:

1 Non-allergenic, causing a minimal soft tissue reaction.
2 Strong and fatigue resistant.
3 Resistant to reabsorption, corrosion or deformation.
4 Non-supportive of growth of micro-organisms.
5 Radiolucent.
6 Cheap.
7 Readily available.

Classification

Implants may be classified into:

- Liquids (silicone, collagen preparations, hyaluronic acid preparations)
- Solids (metals, polymers, ceramics).

Liquids

Silicone

- Silicon is an element.
- Silica is silicone oxide and is the main constituent of sand.
- Silicone consists of interlinked silicon and oxygen molecules with methyl, vinyl or phenol side groups.
- Short polymer chains produce a viscous liquid.
- Long polymer chains produce a firmer, cohesive gel.
- Cross-linking of the chains produces solid silicone.
- Silicon is biologically inert but elicits a mild foreign-body reaction with subsequent capsule formation.
- Synovitis can occur when silicone prostheses are used in joint arthroplasty.
- Bioplastique consists of textured silicone-rubber microparticles mixed with water in a hydrogel carrier.

There has been much debate as to whether silicone implantation is associated with an increased risk of developing connective tissue diseases.

- Extensive reviews of the safety of silicone have been performed:
  - In the USA by the Institute of Medicine (IOM) of the National Academy of Science
  - In the United Kingdom by the Independent Review Group.
- Both of these reviews concluded that there was no evidence that silicone implants were responsible for any major diseases.
- The findings of these groups are discussed in more detail in 'Plastic surgery of the breast and chest wall. Breast augmentation', see pp. 177–8.

Collagen preparations

Zyderm 1

- This is made from sterilized, fibrillar bovine collagen.
- It is composed of 95% type 1 collagen and 5% type 3 collagen.
- The collagen concentration is 35 mg/mL.
- It is administered via injection and is used for treating fine, superficial wrinkles.

Zyderm 2

- This has a similar collagen composition to Zyderm 1.
- The collagen concentration is higher, at 65 mg/mL.
- It is used to treat coarser wrinkles.
- Absorption of the water carrier from both Zyderm 1 and Zyderm 2 reduces their injected volume by approximately 30%.
- Soft-tissue defects should therefore be overcorrected initially.

Zyplast

- This is formed by cross-linking the collagen with glutaraldehyde.
- It is firmer than either Zyderm 1 or Zyderm 2.

· It is used to treat deep dermal defects and coarse rhytids.
· Little reabsorption occurs 50 overcorrection is not recommended.

Hyaluronic acid preparations
· A number of preparations, such as Restylane and Perlane, composed of synthetically manufactured hyaluronic acid are now available.
· Average absorption rates are 20%–50% of the original volume by 6 months.
· These preparations are typically injected superficially, to treat wrinkles or increase lip definition.

Solids

Metals

Stainless steel
· Stainless steel is an alloy of iron, chromium and nickel.
· It has a relatively high incidence of corrosion and implant failure.
· Galvanic currents set up between screws and the plates can result in corrosion.

Vittalium
· Vittalium is an alloy of chromium, cobalt and molybdenum.
· It has a higher tensile strength than either stainless steel or titanium.

Titanium
· Titanium is a pure material and not an alloy.
· It is more malleable and less prone to corrosion than either stainless steel or vittalium.
· In addition, it is less likely to produce an artefact on MRI or CT scanning.

Gold
· Gold is resistant to corrosion but has a low tensile strength.
· It is used primarily as an upper-eyelid weight to facilitate eye closing in facial palsy.

Polymers

Polyurethane
· This polymer induces an intense foreign-body reaction followed by tissue adhesion.
· Breast implants covered with polyurethane foam have a low rate of capsular contracture.
· Breakdown products of polyurethane include toluene-diamine dimers.
· Concern over the risk of carcinogenesis from the build-up of these dimers has resulted in withdrawal of these breast implants.

Fluorocarbons

- Bonding between fluorine and carbon results in an extremely stable biomaterial.
- No human enzyme can break the bond between the two substances.

Proplast 1

- This is a black composite of Teflon and carbon.
- It is used for facial bony augmentation.

Proplast 2

- This is a white composite of Teflon and aluminium oxide.
- It is used for more superficial augmentation.
- A high rate of complications (infection, extrusion, etc.) with proplast temporomandibular joint (TMJ) implants resulted in its withdrawal from the market in the USA.

Goretex

- This is a sheet of expanded polytetrafluoroethylene (PTFE).
- It is soft and very strong.
- PTFE has been used as a vascular prosthesis since 1975.
- Goretex has been approved for facial implantation in the USA since 1994.

Polyethylene

- This material has a simple carbon chain structure and, unlike the fluorocarbons, does not contain fluorine.
- It is available in three grades:
  1. Low density
  2. High density
  3. Ultra-high molecular weight.
- Medpor is high-density, porous polyethylene.
- It is commonly used for augmenting the facial skeleton.
- It elicits very little foreign-body reaction.
- Some soft tissue ingrowth does occur—this acts to stabilize the implant.
- Medpor implants are available in a variety of preformed shapes.
- Ultra-high molecular weight polyethylene is used in the fabrication of load-bearing orthopaedic implants.

Polypropylene

- Polypropylenes have a similar structure to polyethylenes.
- They differ by containing a methyl group instead of a hydrogen atom in each unit of the polymer chain.
- Marlex polypropylene mesh has high tensile strength and allows early tissue ingrowth.

Methylmethacrylate

- This is a self-curing acrylic resin.
- It is used for:
  - Securing artificial joint components
  - Craniofacial bone augmentation
  - Fabrication of gentamicin-impregnated beads.
- It is available in two forms:
  1. As a paste that dries, forming a solid block
  2. As preformed implants.
- Methylmethacrylate elicits an exothermic reaction during drying.
- When used for calvarial remodelling, it is important to cool the methylmethacrylate to avoid soft-tissue burn.

Cyanoacrylate

- This is the main constituent of superglue.
- It is a strong, biodegradable tissue adhesive.
- Clinically, it is used for:
  - Opposing skin edges
  - Securing skin grafts
  - Securing nails to their underlying beds.
- It is particularly useful for repairing simple lacerations in children, as it avoids the pain associated with suturing.

Ceramics

Hydroxyapatite

- This is the major inorganic constituent of bone.
- It is produced by corals and is available in block, granule or cement form.
- Hydroxyapatite is osseoconductive, allowing creeping substitution.
- It has no osseoinductive or osteogenic properties.
- BoneSource is hydroxyapatite cement.
- When mixed with water and a drying agent, this material forms a paste which rapidly hardens.
- Clinically it is used for:
  - Inlay calvarial remodelling
  - Onlay calvarial remodelling
  - Augmentation of the facial skeleton.
- Inlay calvarial remodelling is the replacement of the full thickness of the skull.
- Onlay calvarial remodelling is the replacement of a portion of the outer thickness of the skull.

Other ceramics

Other alloplastic ceramics include:

- Calcium sulfate (plaster of Paris)
- Calcium phosphate.

Wound dressings

There is little concrete evidence that any one dressing is better than another. The ideal wound dressing should:

1 Protect the wound physically
2 Be non-irritant
3 Remove necrotic material
4 Promote epithelialization
5 Promote granulation
6 Be cheap and readily available.

Classification

Wound dressings can be broadly classified into the following groups.

Low-adherent dressings

- Melolin is gauze with polyethylene backing.
- Inadine is a rayon mesh impregnated with povidone-iodine.
- Paraffin gauze-based dressings include:
  - Jelonet
  - Bactigras (paraffin gauze impregnated with chlorhexidine).

Semipermeable films

- Semipermeable films are:
  - Permeable to gases and vapour
  - Impermeable to liquids and bacteria.
- Omniderm is a polyurethane film without an adhesive backing.
- Opsite and Tegaderm are polyurethane films with adhesive backing.

Hydrogels

- Hydrogels are composed of a starch-polymer matrix which swells to absorb moisture.
- They promote autolysis of necrotic material and are principally used to debride wounds.

Hydrocolloids

- This dressing is composed of a hydrocolloid matrix backed with adhesive.
- It physically protects the wound while absorbing fluid and maintaining a moist environment.
- Examples include:
  - Granuflex
  - Duoderm.

Alginates

- These substances are derived from seaweed.
- They contain calcium which activates the clotting cascade when exchanged with sodium within the wound.

- They are very absorbent and become gelatinous upon absorbing moisture.
- Examples include:
  - Sorbisan
  - Kaltostat.

Synthetic foams
- These foams are usually used in concave wounds.
- They conform to the cavity, obliterating dead space.
- They are suitable for heavily exudating wounds.
- An example of this type of dressing is Lyofoam.

Vacuum-assisted wound closure
- It has recently been discovered that the application of suction to a wound speeds its healing.
- The mechanism by which this occurs is uncertain.
- Possible mechanisms include:
  - A direct suction effect on the wound edges and base, pulling the wound inwards.
  - An increase in the rate of angiogenesis and the formation of granulation tissue.
  - A reduction in the concentration of tissue metalloproteinases.
  - A decrease in the bacterial contamination of the wound.
  - A decrease in the interstitial fluid content of the wound.
- Suction is applied to the wound in the following manner.
  1 The wound is covered with a non-adherent, sponge dressing containing the end of a suction tube.
  2 The wound is then sealed with a semipermeable, adhesive film.
  3 Intermittent or continuous suction is then applied to the wound from a specifically designed machine.
- Suction pressures are usually set at approximately 120 mmHg for acute wounds and 50–70 mmHg for chronic wounds.

Sutures and suturing

Suturing
- The skin edges should always be everted when suturing is complete.
- This results in:
  - Better dermal apposition
  - Improved healing
  - A finer final scar.
- Most wounds are closed by first opposing the skin edges with a dermal suture.
- This reduces the tension on the subsequent cutaneous suture and helps to limit stretching of the wound.

Dermal suture

· The dermal suture should enter the deep reticular dermis on the incised edge of the wound.
· It should then pass superficially into the papillary dermis.
· The knot should be tied deeply to prevent subsequent exposure of the suture.
· This method of suture placement produces good apposition and eversion of the skin edges.
· If one side of the wound is longer than the other, the suture should be passed more superficially on the long side and deeper on the short side.
· Passing the suture in this way tends to gather up the longer side, allowing neater wound closure.

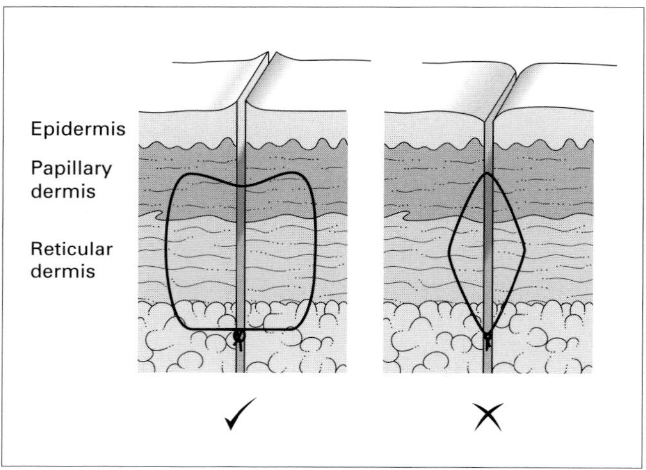

Cutaneous suture

· The aim of this suture is to accurately appose and evert the skin edges.
· The following may be helpful in achieving this.
  · When viewed in a cross-section, the suture passage should be triangular-shaped with its base located deeply—this will evert the wound edges.
  · A triangular-shaped suture passage with the base located superficially tends to invert the wound edges.

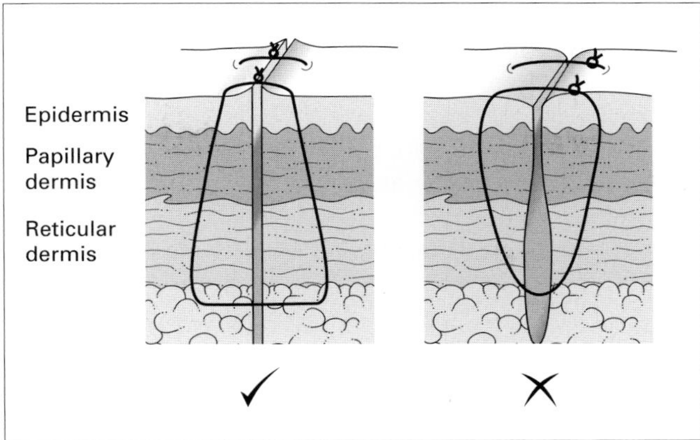

- If one of the wound edges lies lower than the other, the suture should be passed through the cut edge of the skin low on that side ('low-on-the-low').
- If one of the wound edges lies higher than the other, the suture should be passed through the dermis high on that side ('high-on-the-high').
- Passing the suture in this way acts to flatten out any vertical step between the wound edges and ensures that the sides are on a level plane.
- Fine adjustments can be made by changing the side on which the knot lies (the knot will tend to raise the side on which it lies).

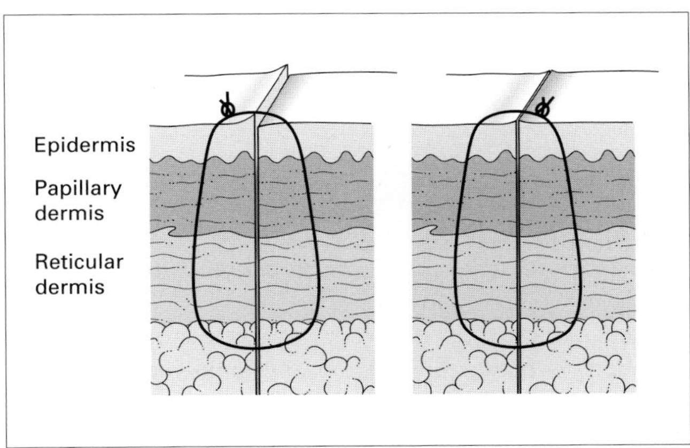

Intradermal skin suturing

- This technique is often incorrectly called subcuticular suturing.
- The suture passes through the dermis, not under the skin.
- The suture should enter deeply from deep in the reticular dermis on the incised skin edge.
- It should then pass more superficially into the papillary dermis at a level just deep enough to avoid puckering of the skin.

- This results in:
  - Eversion of the skin edges
  - Burying of the knot deeply so that it is unlikely to protrude through the skin, forming a stitch abscess.
- Sutures that retain their strength for a significant amount of time, such as a polydioxanone suture (PDS), should be used in areas prone to scar stretching, such as the back.
- Sutures that elicit a minimal tissue reaction, such as monocryl, should be used in the face.

Suture materials

Sutures are either: (i) absorbable or non-absorbable; (ii) synthetic or natural; or (iii) braided or monofilament.

Absorbable sutures

Catgut

- Catgut is derived from the submucosal layer of sheep intestine.
- It elicits a significant inflammatory response.
- Its absorption is unpredictable.
- It loses its strength by 8–9 days.
- It is absorbed by 1 month.
- A decreased rate of absorption occurs if the suture is chromatized (chromic catgut).
- Clinically catgut is usually used as:
  - A mucosal suture
  - A dermal suture in the face
  - A skin suture in children.

Polyglycolic acid

- Dexon is a synthetic suture composed of polyglycolic acid.
- It is degraded by hydrolization.
- It loses its strength by 21 days and is absorbed by 90 days.

Polyglactin 910

- Vicryl is a braided synthetic suture composed of polyglactin 910.
- It loses its strength by 21 days and is absorbed by 90 days.
- Its braided nature may make it more prone to bacterial colonization than monofilament alternatives.
- It may provoke a significant inflammatory reaction and some recommend that it is not used as a dermal suture in the face.

Poliglecaprone 25

- Monocryl is a monofilament synthetic suture composed of poliglecaprone 25.
- It has similar absorption characteristics to vicryl.
- Its monofilament composition may make it less prone to bacterial colonization.

Polydioxanone

- PDS is a monofilament synthetic suture composed of polydioxone.
- It is absorbed more slowly than either vicryl, monocryl or dexon.
- It loses its strength by 3 months and is absorbed by 6 months.
- It is primarily used as a dermal suture in areas prone to developing stretched scars.

Non-absorbable sutures

- Non-absorbable sutures are generally used as:
  - Cutaneous stitches which will need to be removed
  - Deep stitches to provide permanent tissue fixation.
- Non-absorbable sutures may be natural or synthetic.

Natural

- Silk
- Cotton.

Synthetic

- Polyamide
  - Nylon
  - So-named because it was developed jointly in **N**ew **Y**ork and **LON**don.
- Polypropylene
  - Prolene.
- Stainless steel.

Tissue expansion

- Tissue expansion, by techniques such as neck lengthening, has been practised since ancient times.
- More recently, in 1957, Neuman described tissue expansion for therapeutic purposes.
- Since then, it has been popularized by authors such as Radovan.

Mechanisms

- Approximately 70% of tissue gain is due to stretch and 30% due to growth.
- As tissue stretches, it relaxes, and less force is required to keep it stretched—this is known as stress relaxation.
- Tissue creep is the time-dependent plastic deformation of any material in response to constant stress.
- Tissue creep occurs because of disruption of elastin fibres.
- If a plastic bag is stretched, it stays in a stretched state—this is tissue creep.
- The initial force required to stretch a plastic bag is greater than that needed to maintain it stretched—this is stress relaxation.

Changes

Tissue-expanded skin is characterized by the following changes.

The epidermis

The thickness of the epidermis usually increases but can remain the same as in unexpanded skin.

The dermis

- The thickness of the dermis decreases as the skin is expanded.
- The collagen fibres within the dermis realign along the lines of tension during expansion.

The mitotic rate of the skin

The mitotic rate of skin increases with the application of traction.

The skin appendages and nerves

- These become increasingly separated from one another during expansion.
- Hair density is therefore reduced in expanded skin.

The subcutaneous tissue, muscle and bone

Pressure effects exerted by the expander may lead to localized atrophy of the surrounding tissue.

Microscopic appearance of the expander capsule

Paysk has described four zones within the capsule surrounding an expander.

1 The inner zone is a fibrin layer containing macrophages.
2 The central zone contains elongated fibroblasts and myofibroblasts.
3 The transitional zone is composed of loose collagen fibers.
4 The outer zone contains blood vessels and collagen.

Advantages

Advantages of tissue expansion include the following.

- Reconstruction with tissue of a similar colour and texture to that of the donor defect
- Reconstruction with sensate skin containing skin appendages
- Limited donor-site deformity.

Insertion and placement of expanders

Tissue expanders can be inserted through a wide variety of incisions.

- These may be local or remote.
- Expander insertion through a remote, radially orientated incision is associated with the lowest complication rate.
- Expanders can be placed below or above the fascia.
- Subcutaneous placement is usually preferred in the face and trunk.
- Subfascial placement is usually preferred in the forehead and scalp.

Contraindications

Ideally, tissue expanders should not be inserted:

- In the vicinity of an immature scar
- In the presence of infection
- In irradiated tissue
- Under skin grafts.

Design of expanders

Tissue expanders are essentially expandable, saline-filled bags. They differ from one another in the following ways.

Shape

- Oval
- Rectangular
- Round
- Square
- Crescentic (croissant-shaped)
  - Croissant-shaped expanders may result in shorter donor defects.
  - This is because expansion principally occurs over the central portion of the expander.

Size

- Base dimensions
- Projection when inflated.

Location of the port

- Integrated ports form part of the shell of the expander.
- Remote ports are attached to the expander by a filling tube.
- Remote ports can be placed subcutaneously or externally.

Envelope composition

- The shell of an expander can have a smooth or textured surface.
- The shell is usually of a uniform thickness and compliance.
- Variations in shell thickness and compliance can be used to produce preferential expansion in a certain direction or directions.
- Expanders may or may not have a stiff backing bonded onto their shell.

Timing and length of expansion

Tissue expansion can be performed by the following methods.

Intra-operative expansion

Examples of this method of tissue expansion include:

- Sustained traction applied to the tissue by skin hooks or other instruments
- Tissue expansion with a Foley catheter
- Sureclosure devices.

Rapid expansion

- The rationale behind this technique is that most tissue creep and growth occurs in the first 2 days following expansion.
- Some authorities therefore recommend inflation of the expander every 2–3 days.

Conventional expansion

- Most tissue expanders are inflated weekly.
- This allows sufficient time for the tissues to stabilize between expansions.
- Expansion is stopped when the amount of tissue gained is sufficient to permit adequate reconstruction. This can be estimated by:
  - Recording the dimensions of the tissue over the expander from fixed points before it is inflated.
  - Comparing these measurements to the dimensions of the tissue over the expander when it is inflated.
  - Comparing the tissue gain to the dimensions of the defect.

Complications

- The complications of tissue expansion include:
  - Haematoma
  - Infection
  - Exposure of the expander
  - Extrusion of the expander
  - Pain
  - Neurapraxia
  - Pressure effects on surrounding tissue.
- Minor complications are those that do not result in the termination of the procedure.
- Major complications are those that do result in the termination of the procedure.

Further reading

Adzick NS, Lorenz HP. Cells, matrix, growth factors and the surgeon. The biology of scarless fetal wound repair. *Ann Surg* 1994; **220** (1): 10–8

Austad ED, Thomas SB, Paysk K. Tissue expansion: dividend or loan? *Plast Reconstr Surg* 1986; **78** (1): 63–7.

Borges AF. Relaxed skin tension lines (RSTL) versus other skin lines. *Plast Reconstr Surg* 1984; **73** (1): 144–50.

Borges AF. W-plasty. *Ann Plast Surg* 1979; **3** (2): 153–9.

Cormack GC, Lamberty BGH. A classification of fascio-cutaneous flaps according to their pattern of vascularity. *Br J Plast Surg* 1984; **37** (1): 80–7.

DeLacure MD. Physiology of bone healing and bone grafts. *Otolaryngol Clin North Am* 1994; **27** (5): 859–74.

Gordh M, Alberius P, Johnell O *et al.* Effects of rhBMP-2 and ostoepromotive membranes on experimental bone grafting. *Plast Reconstr Surg* 1999; **103** (7): 1909–18.

Hauben DJ, Baruchin A, Mahler A. On the history of the free skin graft. *Ann Plast Surg* 1982; **9** (3): 242–5.

Holmes RE. Alloplastic implants. In: McCarthy JG (ed). *Plastic Surgery*. Philadelphia: WB Saunders, 1990: 698–703.

Jackson IT. *Local Flaps in Head and Neck Reconstruction.* St Louis: Mosby, 1985.

Johnson TM, Lowe L, Brown MD, *et al.* Histology and physiology of expanded tissue. *J Dermatol Surg Oncol* 1993; **19** (12): 1074–8.

Robson MC, Mustoe TA, Hunt TK. The future of recombinant growth factors in wound healing. *Am J Surg* 1998; **176** (2A Suppl): 80S–82S.

Rohrich RJ, Zbar RI. A simplified algorithm for the use of the Z-plasty. *Plast Reconstr Surg* 1999; **103** (5): 1513–7.

Ryan TJ. Exchange and the mechanical properties of skin: oncotic and hydrostatic forces control by blood supply and lymphatic drainage. *Wound Repair Regener* 1995; **3**: 258–64.

Taylor GI, Palmer JH. The vascular territories (angiosomes) of the body: experimental study and clinical applications. *Br J Plast Surg* 1987; **40** (2): 113–41.

Zins JE, Whitaker LA. Membranous versus endochondral bone: Implications for craniofacial reconstruction. *Plast Reconstr Surg* 1983; **72** (6): 778–85.

Skin and soft-tissue lesions

Benign non-pigmented skin lesions

Skin lesions can be derived from any of the constituents of the skin; these include:

- The epidermis
- The dermis
  - Hair follicles
  - Eccrine glands
  - Sebaceous glands
  - Neural tissue.
- Cysts
  - Epidermoid cysts
  - Pilar cysts
  - Milia
  - Xanthalasma.

Skin lesions of epidermal origin

Basal cell papillomas

- This common lesion is also known as a seborrheic keratosis.
- It is a greasy plaque-like lesion usually found on the torso of elderly patients.
- If indicated, treatment is by curettage.

Squamous papillomas

- These common skin lesions are also known as 'skin tags' and 'acrochordons'.
- Treatment is by excision.

Viral warts

- These lesions are caused by the human papilloma virus.
- Treatment is with cryotherapy or curettage.

Actinic keratosis

- These are scaly crusted areas that occur in the sun-exposed areas of the elderly.
- Approximately 20–25% develop into squamous cell carcinomas (SCCs).

Keratotic horns

- This is a hard protruding lump of cornified material.
- An actinic keratosis (AK), or occasionally an SCC, is usually found at the base of the lesion.

Bowen's disease

- This is a red scaly lesion usually found on the legs of elderly patients.
- Histologically it resembles an SCC.
- The microscopic abnormalities are limited to the epidermis and the lesion is best regarded as an *in situ* SCC.
- These lesions are generally removed as they can progress to form invasive SCCs.
- Non-operative treatment with argotherapy has produced good results.

Keratoacanthoma

- Keratoacanthomas (KAs) enlarge rapidly to form nodules with a central keratotic core.
- KAs typically involute without treatment leaving a depressed scar.
- Histologically, these lesions are difficult to differentiate from SCCs.
- Some authorities maintain that they are, in fact, well-differentiated SCCs rather than a distinct clinical entity.
- Ferguson–Smith syndrome is a condition linked to a single gene mutation in the West of Scotland over 200 years ago.
- The condition has the following characteristics.
  - Autosomal dominant inheritance
  - The development of multiple self-healing epitheliomas which look and behave like KAs.

Skin lesions of dermal origin

Lesions derived from the hair follicles

Trichoepithelioma

- These are translucent pinky–white nodules.
- They are often located around the nose and mouth.

Trichofolliculoma

- These are nodules with a central pore which often contains a collection of white hairs.
- Histologically, the lesions resemble basal cell carcinomas (BCCs).
- However, unlike BCCs, they contain keratin-filled macrocysts.

Tricholemmoma

- These are small warty papules.
- Cowden's syndrome is characterized by the following.
  - Multiple facial tricholemmomas
  - Keratoses on the palms and soles
  - Oral polyps
  - The development of breast cancer in 50% of patients.

Pilomatrixoma

- This lesion is also known as a calcifying epithelioma of Malherbe.
- It presents as a hard subcutaneous nodule, typically located on the face of children.
- Treatment is by excision.

Lesions derived from the eccrine glands

Eccrine poroma

These lesions are relatively common and present as small nodules on the palm and the sole.

Cylindroma

- These pink lesions usually occur on the scalps of the elderly.
- Large or multiple lesions are known as 'turban tumours'.

Syringoma

These small, firm, skin-coloured nodules typically occur on the eyelid and chest.

Lesions derived from the sebaceous glands

Sebaceous hyperplasia

- These small yellowish lesions are usually found on the face.
- Clinically, they can be confused with BCCs.
- Severe sebaceous hyperplasia of the nose is known as a rhinophyma.

Sebaceous adenomas

These small smooth papules usually occur on the scalp of the elderly.

Sebaceous naevi

- This lesion is also known as a sebaceous naevus of Jadassohn and an organoid naevus.
- It is normally present at birth but usually enlarges and becomes raised in puberty due to hyperplasia of the sebaceous glands.
- These lesions are usually removed as they have a 20–30% chance of malignant transformation.

· Malignant transformation is usually into a BCC or, less commonly, into a mixed appendigeal tumour.

Lesions derived from neural tissue

Neurofibroma

- These skin-coloured nodules are composed of neural tissue and keratin.
- Neurofibromatosis or von Recklinghausen's disease consists of:
  - Multiple cutaneous neurofibromas
  - Five or more café-au-lait patches >1.5 cm in diameter
  - Axillary freckling
  - Lisch nodules on the iris (ocular neurofibromatosis).
- Neurofibromatosis has been classified into many subtypes.
- Of these types, 1 and 2 are the most important:
  - *Type 1*: the most common type consists of the features listed above
  - *Type 2*: associated with the development of neurofibromas within the central nervous system.
- Plexiform neurofibromas are large infiltrative lesions usually found in the head or neck region.
- Wound complications are common following their excision.

Cysts

Epidermoid cysts

Superficial cysts can be caused by:

- Trauma
  - Implantation dermoids, caused by trapping of a segment of epidermis within the dermis.
- Entrapment of the epidermis during facial development
  - These cysts are usually located in a submuscular plane towards the outer corner of the eye.
  - In this location, they are known as angular dermoids.
  - Central dermoids may occur anywhere between the forehead and nasal tip.
  - Care is required in treating central dermoids as they may have deep intracranial extensions.
  - Preoperative radiological assessment is advised prior to surgery.
- Unknown aetiology
  - These are the most common superficial cysts.
  - They classically present as firm subcutaneous swellings attached to the skin.
  - They often have an overlying punctum and are frequently located in the cheek region.
  - Pilar cysts are similar to epidermoid cysts but occur on the scalp.
  - Epidermoid cysts are sometimes incorrectly called sebaceous cysts.
  - Their wall is composed of stratified squamous epithelium and they contain keratinized material as well as sebum secreted by sebaceous glands.

- Treatment is by excision of the cyst together with the overlying punctum.
- Every effort should be made to completely remove the lesion as a recurrent cyst can reform from residual segments.
- Gardener's syndrome consists of multiple epidermoid cysts associated with:
  - Osteomas of the jaw
  - Polyposis coli.

Milia

- Milia are small intra-epidermal cysts.
- They usually occur on the cheeks.
- Treatment is by simple needle enucleation.

Xanthelasma

- These lesions represent an accumulation of lipid within the skin.
- They are usually located around the eyes.
- Treatment involves excision.
- Care must be taken not to cause an ectropion and vertical rather than horizontal excisions may be indicated in some cases.

Benign pigmented skin lesions

Structure and function of melanocytes

- Melanocytes are derived from the neural crest.
- They are spindle-shaped clear cells which contain a dark nucleus and possess dendritic processes.
- Melanin is synthesized within melanocytes from the aminoacid tyrosine via the intermediate DOPA.
- Melanin accumulates in vesicles within melanocytes.
- These vesicles are known as melanosomes.
- Melanosomes are distributed to the surrounding cells via the long dendritic processes of the melanocyte.
- The cells surrounding the melanocytes often contain more melanin than the melanocytes themselves.
- The number of melanocytes does not vary between races.
- The increased pigmentation of darker races is due to increased production of melanin.
- Melanin production is stimulated by sunlight and the pituitary hormone, melanocyte-stimulating hormone (MSH).

Naevus cells

- When melanocytes leave the epidermis and enter the dermis they become naevus cells.
- These cells differ from melanocytes in the following ways.

- They are round rather than spindle shaped.
- They do not have dendritic processes.
- They tend to congregate in nests.

Melanocytic lesions

- Melanocytic lesions may be benign or malignant.
- Malignant melanocytic lesions are known as malignant melanomas.
- Benign melanocytic lesions can be subdivided into those containing naevus cells and those containing melanocytes.
- Naevus cell naevi are either:
  - Congenital; or
  - Acquired.
- Melanocytic naevi originate in either:
  - The epidermis; or
  - The dermis.

Classification of melanocytic naevi

Naevus cell naevi

- Congenital
  - Giant hairy naevus (GHN)
  - Non-GHN
- Acquired
  - Junctional naevus
  - Compound naevus
  - Intradermal naevus
- Special naevi
  - Spitz naevus
  - Dysplastic naevus
  - Halo naevus.

Melanocytic naevi

- Epidermal
  - Ephelis
  - Lentigo
  - Café-au-lait patch
  - Becker's naevus
  - Albright's syndrome
- Dermal
  - Blue naevus
  - Mongolian blue spot
  - Naevus of Ota
  - Naevus of Ito.

Congenital naevus cell naevi

Giant hairy naevi

- To classify as a GHN, lesions have to:
  - Be >20 cm in diameter in the adult, or
  - Cover >5% of the body surface area (BSA).
- The lifetime risk of malignant change within a GHN is probably in the region of 2–4%, although figures of up to 40% have been reported.
- Melanomas arising within a GHN are said to have a worse prognosis than other melanomas.
- Leptomeningeal melanosisis associated with GHN carries a very poor prognosis.
- The best method of treating GHN is controversial.
- Some authorities maintain that the pigment is located superficially in the early neonatal period and thereafter becomes deeper.
- They therefore advocate removal of the lesion early in life.
- This can be performed by:
  - Excision
  - Dermabrasion
  - Curettage
  - Laser ablation.
- Surgical treatment of a GHN in the neonatal period can result in significant morbidity due to blood loss.
- Superficial removal of the lesion can result in the development of residual black areas in later life; these can result in a leopard-skin type appearance.
- It is debatable whether superficial excision reduces the risk of malignant transformation.
- Some authors advocate excision of the lesion during the early childhood years.
- The resultant defect can be reconstructed by one of the following means.
  - Wide undermining and direct closure
  - Tissue expansion
  - Skin grafting.
- Some authors advise against prophylactic surgery for GHN.
- They recommend regular observation with prompt excision of any abnormal areas.
- Because of the relative lack of prospective data on the incidence of malignant change, the optimum method of treating these lesions is not well defined.

Non-giant hairy naevi

- These lesions are usually managed by excision in the early childhood years.
- Reconstruction may require tissue expansion, local flaps or skin grafting.

Acquired naevus cell naevi

- These lesions are rare in infancy.
- Their incidence increases steadily during childhood, sharply during adolescence, more slowly in early adulthood and plateaus in middle age.
- Acquired naevus cell naevi are subdivided into the following groups.

Junctional naevi

· These flat, smooth and irregularly pigmented lesions are usually found in the young.

· They are composed of nests of naevus cells clustered around the epidermal–dermal junction.

Compound naevi

· These are round, well-circumscribed, slightly raised lesions.

· They consist of nests of naevus cells clustered at the epidermal–dermal junction extending into the dermis.

Intradermal naevi

· These are dome-shaped lesions which may be non-pigmented or hairy.

· They tend to occur in adults and are composed of nests of naevus cells clustered within the dermis.

Special naevus cell naevi

Spitz naevi

· These lesions are also known as juvenile melanomas and epitheloid cell naevi.

· They usually present in early childhood as firm reddish-brown nodules.

· Histologically, they have a very similar appearance to melanoma.

· Treatment is by excision with a narrow margin.

Dysplastic naevi

· Dysplastic naevi have:
  · An irregular outline
  · Patchy pigmentation
  · A diameter >5 mm.

· Atypical naevus syndrome is said to exist if >100 dysplastic naevi are present in one patient.

· These lesions are discussed further in the melanoma section (see p. 69).

Halo naevi

· A halo naevus is surrounded by a depigmented area of skin.

· They are relatively common in older children and teenagers.

· Halo naevi tend to regress leaving a small scar.

· Antimelanoma antibodies have been detected in some patients with halo naevi.

· Treatment is expectant.

Epidermal melanocytic naevi

Ephelis

· An ephelis is also known as a freckle.

· It contains a normal number of melanocytes.

· The pigmentation of the lesion is due to increased production of melanin by the melanocytes.
· These lesions are said to disappear in the absence of sunlight.

Lentigo
· These lesions contain an increased number of melanocytes.
· They persist in the absence of sunlight.
· Three types of lentigo are recognized.
  1 Lentigo simplex, which occurs in the young and middle aged
  2 Lentigo senilis, which occurs in the elderly
  3 Solar lentigo, which occurs after sun exposure.

Café-au-lait patch
· This is a pale-brown patch.
· Five or more such lesions >1.5 cm in diameter are required to support a diagnosis of neurofibromatosis.

Becker's naevus
· This is a dark patch on the shoulder.
· It normally appears during adolescence and may become hairy.

Albright's syndrome
This syndrome consists of:
· Pigmented skin lesions
· Fibrous dysplasia
· Precocious puberty.

Dermal melanocytic naevi
These lesions are characterized by the presence of melanocytes within the dermis.

Blue naevus
· These naevi appear as round areas of blue–black discoloration.
· They are thought to result from arrested migration of melanocytes bound for the dermal–epidermal junction.

Mongolian blue spot
· This lesion is characterized by blue–grey pigmentation over the sacrum.
· It is said to be present in 90% of Mongolian infants.

Naevus of Ota
· This lesion is characterized by bluish pigmentation of the sclera and the adjacent periorbital skin.
· The pigmentation is caused by intradermal melanocytes.
· The condition is uncommon in Caucasians but prevalent among Japanese.

Naevus of Ito

- This lesion is characterized by blue–grey discoloration in the shoulder region.
- The pigmentation is caused by intradermal melanocytes.
- The condition is rare in Caucasians but common among Japanese.

Malignant non-pigmented skin lesions

Incidence

Non-pigmented skin cancer is the most common malignancy in the Western world.

Aetiology

Non-melanocytic skin cancer can be caused by the following.

Premalignant conditions

- Bowen's disease
- AKs
- Sebaceous naevi
- Leukoplakia
- Erythroplakia.

Radiation

- UVB and possibly UVA are associated with the development of skin malignancy.
- Radiation exposure from early x-ray machines.

Immunosuppression

- Immunosuppression hampers cell-mediated immunity.
- This results in a reduction in the number and activity of natural killer (NK) cells.

Chronic wounds

- SCCs arising in an area of chronic inflammation are known as 'Marjolin's ulcers'.
- They classically present as unhealed or broken-down areas within an old burn.

Toxins

Toxins known to cause non-melanocytic skin cancer include:

- Soot—historically, there was a high incidence of scrotal cancer in chimney sweeps.
- Arsenic—Bell's Asthma Medicine and Fowler's solution are two medicinal substances that are now known to contain arsenic.

Genetic

Xeroderma pigmentosa

- This condition occurs due to a deficiency of the enzyme thiamine dimerase.
- Thiamine absorbs UV light and forms dimers.
- These dimers cannot be broken down due to the enzyme deficiency.

- The resultant build-up of thiamine dimers induces defects in the structure of DNA.
- This in turn initiates carcinogenisis.

2

Albinism
- Albinism is characterized by the absence of melanin.
- The skin of affected patients is particularly sensitive to the carcinogenic action of UVB radiation.

Fair skin
- Fitzpatrick categorized skin pigmentation into the following six types.
  - *Type 1*: white skin which never tans.
  - *Type 2*: pale skin which burns on sun exposure.
  - *Type 3*: light skin which will tan.
  - *Type 4*: skin of a Mediterranean complexion.
  - *Type 5*: skin of an Indian complexion.
  - *Type 6*: black skin.
- Patients with Fitzpatrick type 1 and 2 skin have a higher incidence of skin cancer.

Types of non-melanocytic skin cancer
- BCC
- SCC
- Merkel cell carcinoma
- Sebaceous carcinoma.

Basal cell carcinoma
- BCCs were known as mariner's disease in the 19th century.
- In France it was known as 'cancer des cultivators'.

Incidence
- 95% of all BCCs occur between 40 and 80 years of age.
- 85% occur in the head and neck.
- Over 200 cases of metastatic BCC have been recorded.

Classification
- Ackerman has formulated over 27 descriptive terms for BCCs.
- Clinically, however, BCCs are either localized, superficial or infiltrative.
- Localized
  - Nodular
  - Nodulocystic
  - Micronodular
  - Pigmented.
- Superficial
  - Superficial spreading
  - Multifocal.

- Infiltrative
  - Morpheic/morpheoform.

Of these, nodular, nodulocystic, superficial and morpheic BCCs are the most common and account for >90% of lesions.

Histological appearance

- BCCs are composed of sheets or nests of small round basophilic cells.
- Their characteristic microscopic appearance is of peripheral pallisading.
- This is a single layer of longitudinally alligned cells at the periphery of the main tumour.
- 95% of BCCs are attached to the epidermis at some point.
- The remaining 5% are attached to a hair follicle.

Gorlin's syndrome

This is an autosomal dominant condition characterized by some, or all, of the following.

- Multiple BCCs
- Palmar pits
- Odontogenic cysts
- Bifid ribs
- Calcification of the falx cerebri
- Overdevelopment of the supraorbital ridges
- Learning difficulties.

Treatment

- BCCs are usually excised with a 2–3 mm margin.
- Lesions with indistinct margins require wider excision.
- Approximately 5% of BCCs will be incompletely excised.
- The rate of incomplete excision is higher in areas such as the inner canthus.
- The treatment of incompletely excised BCCs is controversial.
- Some authorities maintain that it is reasonable to observe rather than re-excise laterally incomplete lesions in areas such as the back.
- Others maintain that all incompletely excised lesions should be re-excised.
- A significant number of re-excisions (>50%) will show no residual tumour.
- Sites in which BCCs are particularly prone to deep invasion are:
  - Around the inner canthus
  - Around the alar base
  - Around the external auditory meatus.
- The reasons for this are unclear but may be because:
  - These are the sites of embryonic fusion of the facial process and invasion can proceed down these natural cleavage lines.
  - Excision and reconstruction in these areas is more complicated than in other sites, consequently insufficient resection is more frequent.
- Modalities other than excision used to treat BCCs include:
  - Radiotherapy

- Photodynamic therapy
- Cryotherapy
- Curettage
- Mohs micrographic surgery
- Intralesional administration of interferon (IF) or BCG vaccine.

· Of these, radiotherapy is the most effective and reports suggest this treatment modality has recurrence rates similar to those of surgery.

Squamous cell carcinoma

- SCCs originate in the stratum spinosum of the epidermis.
- The incidence of SCCs is one-quarter of that of BCCs.
- SCCs often occur in areas of abnormal skin containing:
  - Evidence of sun damage
  - Keratin horns
  - AK
  - Areas of leukoplakia
  - Areas of Bowen's disease.

Histological appearance

- Dysplastic epidermal keratinocytes extend down through the basement membrane into the dermis.
- The presence of keratin pearls is characteristic.
- SCCs may be well, moderately or poorly differentiated.
- Bad prognostic indicators include:
  - Increased depth of invasion
  - Vascular invasion
  - Perineural invasion
  - Lymphocytic infiltration.

Clinical behaviour

- SCCs are prone to local recurrence and metastases.
- The risk of recurrence is related to the histological factors listed above.
- Poorly differentiated SCCs have a 28% risk of recurrence.
- Well-differentiated SCCs have a 7% risk of recurrence.
- The overall risk of occult lymph node metastases at the time of presentation is 2–3%.
- Patients should be followed up regularly to check for local and regional recurrence.

Treatment

- Local excision of SCCs is recommended.
- There is little prospective evidence as to the optimum excision margin.
- 0.5–1 cm excision margins are recommended in most cases.

Merkel cell tumour

- Merkel cells are mechanoreceptors of neural crest origin.
- Merkel cell tumours have the worst prognosis of all primary skin neoplasms.

- These tumours are uncommon and usually occur in the elderly.
- 50% occur on head and neck.
- Histologically, Merkel cell tumours resemble a small cell carcinoma (oat-cell carcinoma).
- It is important to perform a chest x-ray to ensure that the lesion is not a secondary deposit from a lung primary.
- Merkel cell tumours are locally aggressive and tend to metastasize.
- Most patients receive post-operative radiotherapy following excision with a wide margin.

Sebaceous carcinoma

- This is an uncommon tumour arising from sebaceous glands.
- Approximately 50% of all tumours occur in the periorbital region.
- Sebaceous carcinomas are prone to both local and distant recurrence.
- Periorbital lesions are associated with a poor prognosis.
- Treatment is by wide local excision.

Malignant melanoma

Malignant melanoma is a tumour of melanocytes.

Incidence

- Melanoma accounts for approximately 3% of all cancers.
- Its incidence has doubled since 1970.
- There is some evidence that the rapid rise in incidence may be levelling off.
- The lifetime risk of a Caucasian living in Queensland, Australia developing melanoma is one in 14.
- The lifetime risk of a Caucasian living in the USA or the UK developing a melanoma is approximately one in 80.

Risk factors

The risk factors for melanoma can be remembered by the mnemonic 'PPARENTS':

- **P**remalignant lesions
- **P**revious melanoma
- **A**ge
- **R**ace
- **E**conomic status
- Atypical **N**aevus syndrome
- Fitzpatrick **T**ype 1 skin
- **S**unburn.

Premalignant lesions

- Approximately 7% of the general population have one or more atypical naevi.
- Atypical naevus syndrome is defined as the presence of over 100 atypical naevi.
- Patients with atypical naevus syndrome are 12 times more likely to develop a melanoma than patients without these lesions.

- Most melanomas occurring in patients with atypical naevus syndrome arise *de novo* and not from pre-existing moles.
- Prophylactic removal of abnormal naevi does not improve survival.
- The overall lifetime risk of developing a melanoma within a GHN is unclear.
- Malignant transformation rates of 2–40% have been reported.

Ultraviolet radiation

- Ultraviolet light is composed of the following wavelengths.
  1. UVA
     - 315–400 nm
     - This wavelength is emitted by most sunbeds.
     - Exposure is thought, but not proved, to increase the risk of developing melanoma.
  2. UVB
     - 280–315 nm
     - This wavelength produces sunburn.
     - UVB exposure is a known risk factor in the development of melanoma.
  3. UVC
     - 200–280 nm
     - This wavelength is mostly filtered out by the ozone layer.
- Melanoma occurs four times more frequently in patients who had episodes of severe sunburn before the 10 years of age.
- Individuals of a higher economic status are more likely to have had episodes of sunburn as a child, due to holidays abroad.

Classification

Melanoma may be classified in the following ways:

- Clinical and histological characteristics
- Breslow thickness
- Clark's level
- TNM staging
- Clinical staging

Clinical and histological characteristics

- Superficial spreading melanoma: 60%
- Nodular melanoma: 30%
- Melanoma arising in lentigo maligna (LM): 7%
- Acral lentiginous melanoma (ALM): <2%
- Amelanotic melanoma: <1%
- Desmoplastic melanoma: <1%
- Multiple primaries.

Breslow thickness

- This is the distance between the granular layer of the epidermis and the deepest part of the melanoma.
- The Breslow thickness is directly related to survival.

Clark's level

This describes the level into which the tumour has infiltrated.

- *Level I*: tumour confined to the epidermis.
- *Level II*: tumour extending into the papillary dermis.
- *Level III*: tumour extending to the junction between the papillary and reticular dermis.
- *Level IV*: tumour extending into the reticular dermis.
- *Level V*: tumour extending into subcutaneous fat.

TNM staging

TNM staging of melanoma is as follows:

- T*is*: *in situ* melanoma
- T1: depth <0.75 mm; Clark II
- T2: depth 0.75–1.5 mm; Clark III
- T3: depth 1.5–4 mm; Clark IV
- T4: depth >4 mm or the presence of satellite lesions within 2 cm of the primary lesion; Clark V
- N1: node <3 cm or <3 in-transit metastases beyond 2 cm from the original lesion
- N2: node >3 cm or >3 in-transit metastases beyond 2 cm from the original lesion
- M0: no known metastases
- M1: distant metastases.

Clinical staging

The following staging system is used for melanoma.

		10-year survival
Stage 1A	T1N0M0	95%
Stage 1B	T2N0N0	90%
Stage 2A	T3N0M0	65%
Stage 2B	T4N0M0	45%
Stage 3A	Any T N1 M0	15–40%
Stage 3B	Any T N2 M0	
Stage 4	Any T, any N M1	5%

- Intransit metastases are located in the subcutaneous tissue between the primary lesion and the regional lymph node basin.
- Satellite lesions are metastases within the skin.

Adverse effects on prognosis

Factors having an adverse effect on prognosis may be divided into: (i) patient factors; (ii) macroscopic features; and (iii) microscopic features.

Patient factors

- Males have a worse prognosis than females.
- The elderly have a worse prognosis than the young.

Macroscopic features

- Lesions on the trunk, scalp, mucosa and perineum have a worse prognosis, as do ulcerated lesions.
- ALM has a poor prognosis.
- Melanomas arising within an LM have a better prognosis even when tumour depth is taken into account.
- Nodular and superficial spreading melanomas have a similar prognosis when tumour depth is taken into account.

Microscopic features

- The Breslow and Clark measurement of a lesion is related to prognosis.
- Factors such as the presence of a lymphocytic infiltrate and signs of regression may influence prognosis.

Diagnosis

- Prompt diagnosis is crucial in the treatment of melanoma.
- MacKie has described a seven point check list to aid the identification of melanomas.
- The presence of any of the following signs increases the likelihood of a lesion being a melanoma.

Major signs

- Change in size
- Change in shape
- Change in colour.

Minor signs

These can be remembered by the mnemonic 'DISC':

- **D**iameter >5 mm
- **I**nflammation
- **S**ensory change (i.e. itch)
- **C**rusting or bleeding.

Treatment

Primary excision

- Excisional biopsy with a 2 mm margin is usually recommended as the primary treatment for lesions suspected of being melanomas.
- Incisional biopsies are acceptable in the following situations:
  - When the clinical diagnosis of melanoma is uncertain
  - When the lesion is large, so that diagnosis can be confirmed before embarking on a major reconstructive procedure
  - Lentigos not amenable to excision and direct closure
  - Possible subungual melanomas.
- Shave biopsy or curettage is not recommended as a primary treatment as it renders subsequent Breslow and Clark staging inaccurate.

- Excision of a lesion with a 2 mm margin and direct closure may not be possible in some cases.
- In such cases, it is sometimes necessary to dress the wound with moist dressings and await the histology report.
- Once histology is available, informed decisions can be made as to the excision margin and optimum method of reconstruction.

Secondary surgery

- Once melanoma has been confirmed histologically, the patient should undergo a wider excision if this has not already been performed.
- Recently, there has been a trend away from extremely wide excisions.
- Excision with narrower margins has been found to have similar rates of local and distant recurrence.
- Recommended excision margins at present are:
  - Melanoma *in situ*
    - Complete excision with a margin of 5–10 mm.
  - Melanomas with a Breslow depth <1 mm
    - Excision with a 1 cm margin.
  - Melanomas with a Breslow depth of maximum 1–2 mm
    - Excision with a minimum margin of 1 cm and a maximum margin 2 cm.
  - Melanomas with a Breslow depth >2 mm
    - Excision with a minimum margin of 1 cm.
- Availability of local tissue and the patient's preference must be taken into account before deciding on the excision margin.
- Once the excision margin has been established, the skin and subcutaneous tissue should be excised vertically.
- All tissue superficial to the deep fascia should then be removed.
- Reconstruction may be performed by one of the following means.
  - Direct closure
  - Skin grafts
  - Flaps.

Treatment of patients with clinically palpable nodes

- Fine needle aspiration (FNA) is usually performed on suspicious nodes.
- An open biopsy is indicated if clinical suspicion remains despite a negative FNA.
- The incision for an open biopsy must not compromise a subsequent block dissection.

Treatment of patients with histologically positive nodes

- These patients should have the following staging investigations.
  - A chest x-ray
  - Liver function tests
  - An ultrasound, CT or MRI of the abdomen and pelvis.
- If the disease is found to be localized to one lymphatic basin, a block dissection should be performed.

Controversies in treatment

Elective lymph node dissection

- There is little evidence that elective lymph node dissection (ELND) dissection confers a survival benefit.
- The Intergroup Melanoma Trial demonstrated some survival benefit of ELND in patients under 60 years of age with intermediate thickness melanomas (Balch *et al.*, 1996).
- This study did not demonstrate an overall survival benefit in the whole group.
- The current recommendation from the Melanoma Study Group (MSG) is that ELND should not be performed outside of a trial.

Sentinel node biopsy

- This technique aims to identify the first draining node (the sentinel node) within a regional lymphatic basin.
- Preoperative lymphoscintigraphy, vital blue dye injection and the use of a gamma camera are used to identify the sentinel node.
- Routine histology identifies one positive cell in 10 000.
- Serial sectioning and immunostaining increases this to one in 100 000.
- The levels of messenger ribonucleic acid (mRNA) tyrosinase measured by the reverse transcription polymerase chain reaction (RTPCR) identifies one cell in 1 000 000.
- Accurate assessment of the sentinel node has the following advantages.
  - It stages the disease.
  - It may help to determine which patients would benefit from a block dissection.
- At present, there is little evidence that sentinel node biopsy improves prognosis.

Important trials

ECOG trial 1684

- This Eastern Co-operative Oncology Group (ECOG) trial demonstrated an improved overall survival in patients with high-risk melanomas treated with high-dose IF alpha 2b.
- The study suggested that IF might have a role as an adjuvant therapy for melanoma.

WHO trial

- *Lancet* 1998; 351: 793–6.
- This study demonstrated no benefit from ELND.

ECOG trial 1690

- This was a follow-on study after ECOG 1684.
- It demonstrated no increase in overall survival for patients with high-risk melanomas treated with high-dose IF alpha 2b.
- This study cast doubt on the use of IF as an adjuvant therapy for melanoma.

***Koops* et al.**

· *J Clin Oncol* 1998; 16: 2906–12.

· This study demonstrated no survival benefit from prophylactic isolated limb perfusion.

Veronesi

· *N Engl J Med* 1988; 318 (18): 1159–1162.

· This study demonstrated no difference between 1 and 3 cm excision margins in patients with melanomas <2 mm in depth.

Balch

· *Ann Surg* 1995; 218: 262–7.

· This study demonstrated that a 2 cm excision margin was adequate for melanomas 1–4 mm in depth.

Sarcoma

Incidence

· Sarcomas account for approximately 1% of all malignant disease.

· 50% of deep sarcomas occur in the lower extremity, the majority of these are in the thigh.

Classification

Sarcomas can be classified by: (i) tissue of origin; (ii) TNMG classification; (iii) stage; and (iv) Enneking classification.

Tissue of origin

Soft-tissue sarcomas arise from the following tissues.

· Smooth muscle—leiomyosarcoma

· Striated muscle—rhabdomyosarcoma

· Fat—liposarcoma

· Blood vessels—angiosarcoma and Kaposi sarcoma

· Lymph channels—lymphangiosarcoma

· Fibrous tissue—fibrosarcoma

· Nerve—malignant schwannoma

· Synovial tissue—synovial sarcoma

· Skin—dermatofibrosarcoma protuberans (DFSP), atypical fibroxanthoma (AFX), malignant fibrous histiocytoma (MFH).

TNMG classification

· T1: tumours <5 cm in diameter

· T2: tumours >5 cm in diameter

· T3: tumours which invade bone, vessel or nerve

· N0: no nodal disease

· N1: nodal disease confirmed histologically

2

- M0: no metastases
- M1: distant metastases
- G1: low-grade tumour
- G2: intermediate-grade tumour
- G3: high-grade tumour.

Stage

- *Stage 1*: T1 or 2, G1 tumours
- *Stage 2*: T1 or 2, G2 tumours
- *Stage 3*: T1 or 2, N1, G3 tumours
- *Stage 4*: T3, M1 tumours.

Enneking's classification

- 1A: low-grade intracompartmental sarcoma
- 1B: low-grade extracompartmental sarcoma
- 2A: high-grade intracompartmental sarcoma
- 2B: high-grade extracompartmental sarcoma
- 3: regional or distant metastases.

Cutaneous sarcomas

These tumours originate in the skin and are listed in order of increasing malignancy.

Dermatofibrosarcoma protuberans

- This tumour typically appears as a slow-growing, red–brown nodule.
- It is most commonly located on the trunk of young men.
- The mean age of presentation is 35 years.
- These tumours rarely metastasize but are prone to local recurrence.
- They should be excised with a wide margin (up to 5 cm).

Atypical fibroxanthoma

- These tumours usually start as small, firm cutaneous nodules.
- They usually occur in the sun-exposed areas of the head and neck.
- They have malignant-looking histology and stain positively for alpha 1 antitrypsin.
- They rarely recur following wide excision.

Malignant fibrous histiocytoma

- These tumours typically present as firm subcutaneous or cutaneous lesions in elderly patients.
- They are prone to local recurrence and occasionally distant metastases.

Angiosarcoma

- This tumour usually occurs on the face and scalp of elderly patients.
- At presentation, it usually extends microscopically beyond its macroscopic margins.
- Angiosarcoma is particularly prone to local recurrence and metastases.

Deep sarcomas

Presentation

- Deeply located sarcomas usually present as a slowly enlarging mass.
- They may also cause:
  - Pressure on surrounding structures
  - Systemic symptoms such as weight loss, malaise and rigors.

Investigation

Investigation is performed to:

- Obtain a histological diagnosis
- Assess the extent of the lesion.

Investigations to assess the extent of the lesion may include:

- X-rays
- MRI scanning
  - Gadolinium enhancement can be added to aid resolution.
- CT scanning
  - This may be useful to assess bony involvement.
- Angiography
  - This may be performed if vessel involvement is suspected clinically.
- Radionuclide imaging
  - This consists of the following three phases:
    1. An arterial phase, which demonstrates arterial inflow into the tumour
    2. A venous phase, which demonstrates venous pooling within the tumour
    3. An osseous phase, which demonstrates bony invasion.
- Biopsy should be performed to obtain an accurate histological diagnosis.
- It is important that this is performed correctly, as an inappropriate biopsy can significantly worsen prognosis.
- The following points are important.
  - Biopsy should only be performed after delineating deep lesions radiologically.
  - FNA or Tru-cut biopsy can be performed.
  - The skin-entry site must be in an area through which the incision for definitive surgery will pass.
  - Incisional biopsies are not generally recommended.
  - The biopsy should ideally be performed in the unit which will carry out the definitive excisional procedure.

Surgical management

- Large deep sarcomas are best managed in specialist units.
- Deeply situated sarcomas are surrounded by a pseudocapsule.
- Simple enucleation results in prohibitively high recurrence rates.
- These tumours should ideally be resected along with one uninvolved anatomical plane in all directions.
- Functional compartmentectomy (preserving at least one muscle within the compartment) should be performed whenever possible.

- The resection should ideally include both the origin and insertion of the muscle in which the tumour occurs.
- If this is not possible, at least 10 cm of muscle should be excised on either side of tumour.
- If the compartment in which the tumour arises is transversed by a major nerve, it should be preserved unless directly infiltrated by tumour.
- In most cases the patient should receive post-operative radiotherapy.

Radiotherapy

- It has recently been recognized that most sarcomas are radiosensitive to varying degrees.
- Ewing sarcomas, for example, are very radiosensitive.
- Liposarcomas are reasonably radiosensitive.
- Post-operative radiotherapy seems to reduce the risk of local recurrence.
- Radiotherapy typically consist of 50 Gy delivered in 25 fractions over 5 weeks.
- Indications for post-operative radiotherapy include:
  - High-grade tumours
  - Incompletely excised tumours
  - Tumours >5 cm in diameter
  - Deep sarcomas in the head and neck region.

Further reading

Balch CM, Soong SJ, Bartolucci AA *et al.* Efficacy of an elective regional lymph node dissection of 1 to 4 mm melanomas for patients 60 years of age and younger. *Ann Surg* 1996; **224** (3): 255–63.

Balch CM, Urist MM, Karakoussis CP *et al.* Efficacy of 2 cm surgical margins for intermediate thickness melanomas 1 to 4 mm. Results of a multi-institutional randomised surgical trial. *Ann Surg* 1993; **218** (3): 262–7.

Brodland DG, Zitelli JA. Surgical margins for excision of primary cutaneous squamous cell carcinoma. *J Am Acad Dermatol* 1992; **27** (2): 241–8.

Hichcock CL, Bland KI, Laney RG *et al.* Neuroendocrine (Merkel cell) carcinoma of the skin. Its natural history, diagnosis and treatment. *Ann Surg* 1988; **207** (2): 201–7.

Jacobs GH, Rippey JJ, Altini M. Prediction of aggressive behaviour in basal cell carcinoma. *Cancer* 1982; **49** (3): 533–7.

Shore RE. Overview of radiation-induced skin cancer in humans. *Intl J Radiat Biol* 1990; **57** (4): 809–27.

Sober AJ, Fitzpatrick TM, Mihm MC. Primary melanoma of the skin: recognition and management. *J Am Acad Dermatol* 1980; **2** (3): 179–97.

Strom SS, Yamamura Y. Epidemiology of nonmelanoma skin cancer. *Clin Plast Surg* 1997; **24** (4): 627–36.

Veronesi U, Cascinelli N. Narrow excision (1cm margin). A safe procedure for thin cutaneous melanoma. *Arch Surg* 1991; **126** (4): 438–41.

3

The head and neck

Embryology

- 'Branchia' is Greek for 'gill'.
- Branchial arches are paired swellings which lie along the developing neck of the embryo.
- In amphibians branchial arches develop into gills.
- Humans have six paired branchial arches.
- The first and second are the most important in facial development.
- The grooves between the arches on their external surfaces are called branchial clefts.
- The grooves between the arches on their inner surfaces are called pharyngeal pouches.
- The branchial cleft between the first and second arches becomes the external auditory meatus.

Derivatives of the first branchial arch

- The first branchial arch contains/gives rise to:
  - Paired maxillary prominences
  - Paired mandibular prominences.
- The following bones form by intramembranous ossification within the maxillary prominence of the first branchial arch.
  - The maxilla
  - The zygoma
  - The squamous portion of the temporal bone.
- The quadrate cartilage lies within the maxillary process of the first branchial arch; it forms the incus and the greater wing of sphenoid bone.

· Meckel's cartilage lies within the mandibular prominence of the first branchial arch; it mostly resorbs, remaining only in its posterior part as the malleus and the condyles of the mandible.
· The body and the ramus of the mandible form by direct ossification of first arch dermal mesenchyme.
· The trigeminal nerve is derived from the first branchial arch.
· The following muscles are supplied by the trigeminal nerve and are derived from the first branchial arch:
  · The muscles of mastication
  · The anterior belly of the digastric
  · Mylohyoid
  · Tensor veli palatini.

Derivatives of the second branchial arch

· The facial nerve is derived from the second branchial arch.
· The following muscles, supplied by the facial nerve, are derived from the second branchial arch:
  · The muscles of facial expression
  · The posterior belly of digastric
  · Stapedius
  · Stylohyoid.

The frontonasal process

· The frontonasal process is formed by proliferation of mesoderm ventral to the forebrain.
· It is not a branchial arch derivative.
· By the 4th week of intra-uterine life, the frontonasal process has developed paired placodes (ectodermal thickenings) on its inferior border.
· The medial part of the placode forms the medial nasal process.
· The lateral part of the placode forms the lateral nasal process.
· Between the two, a depression known as the nasal pit appears; this becomes the nostril.

Facial development

· Facial development mainly occurs between the 4th and 6th weeks of intra-uterine life.
· The face is formed from the five facial prominences:
  · The paired maxillary processes
  · The paired mandibular processes
  · The frontonasal process.
· The medial nasal process fuses with the maxillary process.
· Failure results in cleft lip (CL).
· Bilateral failure of fusion between maxillary processes and medial nasal process results in a bilateral CL.

· The lateral nasal process fuses with the maxillary process at the alar groove.
· Failure of fusion between the lateral nasal process and the maxillary process results in Tessier #3 cleft.
· Failure of fusion between the maxillary and mandibular processes results in Tessier #7 cleft.

The neural crest

· The neural crest lies on either side of the developing notochord.
· It contains pleuripotential ectomesenchymal tissue.
· Cells originating in the neural crest differentiate into their final cell type on reaching their destination.
· Neural crest derivatives include:
  · The endocrine system
  · The melanocytic system
  · Connective tissue
  · Muscle tissue
  · Neural tissue.

Craniofacial surgery

Classification

The American Society of Cleft Lip and Palate recommends the following classification of craniofacial abnormalities: (i) clefts; (ii) synostosis (syndromal or non-syndromal); (iii) hypoplastic conditions; and (iv) hyperplastic and neoplastic conditions.

Clefts

· Craniofacial clefts have a sporadic incidence and occur approximately once in every 25 000 live births.
· The exact aetiology of craniofacial clefting is unclear.
· Possible causes include:
  · Failure of the facial prominences to fuse
  · Lack of mesodermal penetration
  · Intra-uterine compression by amniotic bands.
· There is some overlap between craniofacial clefts and other hypoplastic syndromes.
· Treacher Collins syndrome is a hypoplastic condition affecting the lateral part of the face.
· It is also known as a confluent 6,7,8 cleft as it consists of features found in all three cleft patterns.
· Craniofacial clefts can affect any or all of the layers of the face.
· The soft-tissue defect does not always correspond to the bony abnormality.
· Craniofacial clefts are often associated with hairline markers.
· These are areas of abnormal linear hair growth along the line of the cleft.

Classification

Tessier's classification of craniofacial clefts is commonly used.

- Facial clefts extend downwards from the level of the orbit.
- Cranial clefts extend upwards from the level of the orbit.
- A midline cleft is numbered 0.
- Facial clefts are numbered 1–7.
  - The numbering of facial clefts starts near the midline with the number 1 cleft.
  - Each sequential facial cleft is more lateral than the last.
  - The number 7 facial cleft is the most lateral and extends outwards from the corner of the mouth.
- Cranial clefts are numbered 8–14.
  - The number 8 cleft is the most lateral and extends into the corner of the orbit.
  - Thereafter, each sequential cranial cleft is more medial than the last.
- Facial and cranial clefts can connect with each other.
  - If this occurs, the patterns tend to add up to 14.
- The number 30 cleft is a midline cleft of the lower lip and mandible.

Specific clefts

Cleft 0

- This cleft is also known as median craniofacial dysraphia.
- It occurs due to failure or delay in the closure of the anterior neuropore.
- The cleft extends downwards in the midline through the frontal bone, the midline of the nose, the columella, the lip and the maxilla.
- It may be associated with encephaloceles and hypertelorism.

Cleft 1

- This cleft is also known as paramedian craniofacial dysraphia.
- The cleft passes downwards between the frontal process of the maxilla and the nasal bone.
- It then extends through the maxilla between the incisors.
- The number 1 cleft may be associated with hypertelorism, widening of the nasal bridge and a bifid nasal dome.

Cleft 2

- This is also known as a paranasal cleft.
- Its path passes slightly lateral to that of cleft 2.

Cleft 3

- This is also known as a oculonasal cleft.
- It runs through the nasal and lacrimal bones into the maxilla.
- The medial wall of the orbit and the lacrimal apparatus may be deficient.
- It is often associated with a coloboma (missing segment) of the medial part of the lower eyelid.
- The lower margin of the cleft passes between the lateral incisor and canine.

Cleft 4

- This is also known as the oculofacial 1 cleft.
- It runs downwards medial to the inferior orbital foramen more laterally than cleft 3.
- The medial wall of the maxilla is uninvolved.
- The lower margin of the cleft extends between the lateral incisor and canine.

Cleft 5

- This is also known as the oculofacial 2 cleft.
- It runs lateral to the inferior orbital foramen.
- It may be associated with a central coloboma of the lower eyelid.

Cleft 6

- This cleft passes between the maxilla and the zygoma.
- It may be associated with a coloboma of the lateral lower eyelid.
- It forms part of Treacher Collins syndrome together with the 7 and 8 clefts.

Cleft 7

- This cleft runs between the zygoma and the temporal bone.
- It may extend medially across the cheek into the lateral aspect of the mouth.
- This may result in macrostomia.

Cleft 8

- This cleft passes outwards from the lateral canthus.
- It extends between the zygoma and the temporal bone into the greater wing of the sphenoid.

Clefts 9, 10 and 11

- These start in the supraorbital region.
- Each sequential cleft is more medial than the last.
- These cranial clefts are often associated with the facial clefts 5, 4 and 3.

Clefts 12, 13 and 14

- These are cranial extensions of facial clefts 2, 1 and 0.
- They do not involve the orbit.
- They may be associated with hypertelorism and widening of the cribriform plate.

Cleft 30

- This is a median cleft of the lower lip and mandible.
- It is an inferior extension of cleft 0.
- The cleft may extend into the neck.

Principles of surgery

- Each cleft is unique and surgery should be tailored to the individual defect.
- The following principles apply to most craniofacial clefts.

- The facial skeleton should be reconstructed by:
  - Removing abnormal elements
  - Transposing skeletal components
  - Bone grafting skeletal defects.
- The facial musculature should be reattached to the skeleton in its correct anatomical position
- The soft tissues should be reconstructed with:
  - Local, regional or distant flaps.

Encephaloceles

- These are caused by herniation of the brain or its lining through a defect in the skull.
- The skeletal defect can result from a craniofacial cleft.
- Encephaloceles are classified by their composition into:
  - Meningoceles—contain meninges
  - Meningoencephaloceles—contain meninges and brain
  - Cystoceles—contain meninges, brain and a portion of ventricle
  - Myeloceles—contain a portion of spinal cord.

Synostosis

- Synostosis is premature fusion of one or more sutures in the cranial vault or skull base.
- It occurs approximately once in every 2500 live births.
- Synostosis may occur:
  - As an isolated abnormality, or
  - As part of a syndrome.
- Non-syndromal synostosis is more common and accounts for approximately 90% of cases.
- The majority of synostosis syndromes are autosomal dominant.
- Genetic mutations can be identified in:
  - 70% of patients with Crouzon, Pfeiffer or Saethre–Chotzen syndrome.
  - Almost 100% of patients with Apert's syndrome.

Aetiology

- The location of the primary abnormality is not clear, however three possible sites have been proposed.
  1. Virchow suggested a primary sutural abnormality.
  2. McCarthy suggested a dural abnormality.
  3. Moss suggested abnormality in the skull base.
- Recent advances in molecular genetics suggest that some synostotic syndromes are caused by abnormalities of the fibroblast growth factor receptors 1, 2, and 3 (FGFRs).

Classification

Synostosis is classified by:

- The location of the affected suture or sutures
- The resultant head shape.

- Any of the following sutures may fuse prematurely:
  - The coronal suture
  - The sagittal suture
  - The metopic suture
  - The lambdoid suture.
- Virchow's law states that skull growth occurs parallel to a synostosed suture.
- Each pattern of fusion therefore results in a characteristic skull shape.
  - Synostosis of the sagittal suture results in an elongated keel-shaped skull (scaphocephaly).
  - Synostosis of one coronal suture results in a twisted skull (plagiocephaly).
  - Synostosis of both coronal sutures results in a short skull in a front-to-back direction (brachycephaly), compensatory growth may occur upwards (turricephaly or acrocephaly).
  - Synostosis of the metopic suture results in a triangular-shaped skull (trigonocephaly).
  - Synostosis of one lambdoid suture results in a twisted skull (posterior plagiocephaly).
  - Synostosis of both lambdoid sutures results in a short skull (brachycephaly).
  - Synostosis of multiple sutures leads to a clover-leaf shaped skull (kleeblattschädel).

3

Clinical features

- The most striking feature is abnormal skull shape.
- The patient may also demonstrate signs and symptoms of raised intracranial pressure; these include:
  - Irritability
  - Tense fontanelles
  - Papilloedema
  - Psychomotor retardation
  - Seizures.
- The incidence of raised intracranial pressure (ICP) increases proportionately with the number of involved sutures.
- The incidence of raised ICP in single suture synostosis is approximately 13%.
- The incidence of raised ICP in multiple suture synostosis is approximately 40%.

Positional plagiocephaly

- It is important to differentiate positional plagiocephaly from true plagiocephaly.
- True plagiocephaly is caused by unilateral synostosis of the coronal or lamdoid sutures.
- Positional plagiocephaly is distortion of the skull due to external pressure.
- The incidence of positional plagiocephaly has increased in recent years due to the trend to nurse babies supine to reduce the risks of cot death.

- Babies tend to lie on one side, leading to an external deforming force on the occipital area: this tends to skew the skull in that direction.
- Positional plagiocephaly should be managed non-operatively as it is usually self correcting.
- Clinical features which differentiate positional from true plagiocephaly include:
  - Skull shape
    - The skull is rhomboid shaped in positional plagiocephaly.
    - In true plagiocephaly, one side of the skull does not grow adequately in a front-to-back direction due to synostosis of the coronal suture.
    - This produces a triangular-shaped skull.
    - The base of the triangle lies on the unaffected side.
    - The apex of the triangle lies on the affected side.
  - Ear position
    - In true plagiocephaly, the distance between the lateral orbit and the ear is reduced.
  - Brow shape
    - The brow has an ipsilateral prominence in positional plagiocephaly.
    - It has a contralateral prominence in true plagiocephaly.
  - Cheek position
    - The ipsilateral cheek is prominent in positional plagiocephaly.

Radiological features

- These may consist of primary changes in the radiological appearance of the suture or secondary changes due to abnormal skull growth.
- Primary changes include:
  1 Loss of suture lucency
  2 Loss of sutural interdigitations
  3 Sclerosis of the suture
  4 Raising (lipping) of the suture.
- Secondary changes include:
  1 An abnormal skull shape
  2 A harlequin appearance of the lateral orbit on AP films (this is caused by the superior displacement of the lesser wing of the sphenoid bone)
  3 A copper-beaten appearance of the skull (a sign of raised ICP).

Syndromal synostosis

Synostosis is a feature of the following syndromes.

Crouzon syndrome

- This is also known as acrocephalosyndactyly type 2.
- It is autosomal dominant, affecting approximately one in 15 000 births.
- Clinical features include:
  1 Bicoronal synostosis
  2 Midfacial hypoplasia with significant exorbitism
  3 Normal hands.

Apert's syndrome
- This is also known as acrocephalosyndactyly type 1.
- It occurs once in approximately 160 000 live births.
- Clinical features include:
  1 Bicoronal synostosis
  2 Midface hypoplasia
  3 A small, beaked nose
  4 Class 3 occlusion
  5 Cleft palate (CP) in 20% of cases
  6 Complex syndactyly.
- The hand deformity is classified in the following way:
  - *Class 1*: the little finger and thumb are separate.
  - *Class 2*: only the thumb is separate.
  - *Class 3*: all the fingers are involved in the syndactyly.

Saethre–Chotzen syndrome
- This is also known as acrocephalosyndactyly type 3.
- Clinical features include:
  1 Bicoronal synostosis
  2 A low-set hair line
  3 Ptosis
  4 Small, posteriorly displaced ears
  5 Simple syndactyly of the hands and feet.

Pfeiffer syndrome
- This is also known as acrocephalosyndactyly type 5.
- The facial appearance is similar to that of Apert's syndrome.
- The hallmark feature of this syndrome is the presence of broad toes and thumbs.

Carpenter syndrome
- This is a rare condition.
- Various sutures may be involved.
- Clinical features include:
  1 Partial syndactyly of the fingers
  2 Preaxial polydactyly (see p. 204).

Treatment

Treatment of synostosis may include the following.

Sagittal strip craniectomy
- If performed at an early age this technique can be used to treat isolated sagittal suture synostosis.
- A longitudinal strip of bone over the suture is excised.
- This releases the constriction and allows the underlying brain to expand the skull.

Fronto-orbital advancement

- This operation advances the frontal part of skull.
- It allows anterior skull growth.
- It is usually performed before the child is 1 year of age.

Le Fort 3 osteotomy

- This is performed to correct midface retrusion encountered in syndromal synostosis.
- Advancements are usually limited to about 1 cm.

Skeletal distraction

- This technique has been described relatively recently.
- Osteotomies are made at similar sites to those of a Le Fort 3 advancement (see p. 132).
- A distraction device is then fitted.
- Greater midfacial advancement can be achieved with distraction than by single-stage Le Fort 3 advancement.

Monobloc advancement

- This technique advances the fronto-orbital and Le Fort 3 segments as one block.
- Communication between the cranial and nasal cavities may result in a high infection rate and subsequent increased mortality.

Hypertelorism

- Hypertelorism is an increase in the distance between the bony orbits.
- Hypotelorism is an abnormally short distance between the orbits.
- Hypotelorism can be caused by synostosis of the metopic suture.
- Telecanthus is an increase in the intercanthal distance (ICD).
- In telecanthus, the distance between the bony orbits may be normal.
- Pseudo-telecanthus is the illusion of telecanthus caused by a flat nasal bridge or prominent epicanthal folds.

Classification

- Tessier has classified hypertelorism according to interorbital distance (IOD):
  - *Type 1*: IOD 30–34 mm
  - *Type 2*: IOD 35–39 mm
  - *Type 3*: IOD Over 40 mm.
- Monroe has described an alternate classification based on the configuration of the medial orbital wall.

Causes

- Hypertelorism is not a syndrome itself but a physical finding associated with numerous conditions, including:

- Median and paramedian facial clefts
- Craniofacial syndromes
  - Apert's syndrome
  - Crouzon's syndrome
  - Craniofacial nasal dysplasia.
- Syncipital (frontal or nasofrontal) encephaloceles
- Midline tumours.

Surgical management

The following operations can be used to correct hypertelorism.

- Box osteotomy
  - In this procedure, rectangular osteotomies are made around each orbit.
  - Bone between the rectangular segments is then removed and the orbits are moved medially towards each other.
  - This operation is used in patients with isolated hypertelorism and a normal midface width.
- Facial bipartition
  - In this procedure, the whole facial skeleton is divided vertically in the midline.
  - A central bony segment is then removed and the two lateral segments containing the orbits are moved medially towards each other.

Hypoplastic conditions

Hypoplastic conditions include: (i) hemifacial microsomia; (ii) Treacher Collins syndrome; and (iii) hemifacial atrophy.

Hemifacial microsomia

- This is a congenital condition characterized by the underdevelopment of one side of the face, and is also known as:
  - First and second branchial arch syndrome
  - Otomandibular dysostosis.
- Hemifacial microsomia is relatively common and affects one in 5000 live births.
- Unlike Treacher Collins syndrome, it is usually asymmetrical.
- Goldenhar's syndrome consists of the following triad.
  1 Hemifacial microsomia
  2 Epibulbar dermoids
  3 Vertebral abnormalities.

Classification

The following classifications of hemifacial microsomia have been described.

- 'OMENS' classification
  - This system individually classifies the deformities of the **O**rbits, **M**andible, **E**ar, Facial **N**erve and **S**oft tissue.
- Prozansky classification

- This system classifies the mandibular deformity:
  - *Group 1*: mild mandibular hypoplasia.
  - *Group 2a*: severe mandibular hypoplasia.
  - *Group 2b*: severe mandibular hypoplasia associated with a non-articulating temporomandibular joint (TMJ).
  - *Group 3*: hypoplasia of the ramus of the mandible associated with an absent TMJ.

3

Treatment

Treatment should be individualized to the patient. The following is a general guide to the timing and nature of the surgery.

Before 2 years of age

- Remove any auricular appendages.
- Correct macrostomia with a commissuroplasty.
- Occasional involvement of the fronto-orbital region may require a fronto-orbital advancement.

Between 2 and 6 years of age

- Distraction of the mandibular ramus.
- Prozansky 3 deformities may require formal reconstruction of the mandibular ramus.
- This is usually performed with a costochondral rib graft.

Between 6 and 14 years of age

- Orthodontic treatment.
- Ear reconstruction.
- Soft-tissue augmentation, often by free-tissue transfer.

After 14 years of age

- Bone grafting to deficient areas of the facial skeleton.
- Orthognathic surgery.

Treacher Collins syndrome

- Treacher Collins syndrome is also known as:
  - Franceschetti syndrome
  - Mandibulofacial dysostosis
  - Confluent 6,7,8 cleft.
- It is autosomal dominant affecting between one in 25 000 and one in 50 000 live births.

Clinical features

Treacher Collins syndrome consists of bilateral abnormalities of the first and second branchial arches. Typically, abnormalities are present in the following sites.

Orbit
- Part of the lateral lower eyelid may be absent (coloboma).
- The eye lashes are often absent medially.
- The tarsal plate may be atrophic.
- The lateral canthus may be displaced medially.
- The lacrimal apparatus may be absent.
- Laterally the eyes may slant downwards.

Nose
- This is typically narrow, deviated and hooked.

Cheek
- The zygoma may be hypoplastic or absent.
- A depression may be present between the corner of the mouth and the angle of the mandible.
- This depression runs along the line of a number 7 cleft.

Palate
- A CP may occur.
- If not, the palate is usually highly arched.

Mandible
- The ramus of the mandible is often short.
- The TMJ is often hypoplastic or absent.

Ear
- The ear may be small (microtia) or buried under the skin posterioly (cryptotia).
- Middle ear deformities may include missing ossicles or cavities.

Treatment

The airway
- Patients with Treacher Collins syndrome often have difficulty maintaining their airway.
- This occurs due to a combination of maxillary and mandibular hypoplasia.
- Nursing them in a prone position can often improve their oxygen saturation.
- Tracheostomy may be required in very severe cases.

The zygoma and orbit
- Calvarial bone grafting is often used to augment the orbital floor and zygoma.
- This is usually performed once the child is at least 7 years of age.

The mandible

The mandibular deformity may be corrected with:

- Rib grafts
- Mandibular advancement
- Bimaxillary procedures
- Distraction.

The ear

- Reconstruction of the external ear may be required (see pp. 154–5).
- Hearing deficits can be improved with bone-conducting hearing aids.

Hemifacial atrophy

- This acquired condition is also known as Romberg's disease.
- It is usually unilateral.
- It occurs sporadically and is not associated with a positive family history.
- Its aetiology is unknown but may be due to viral infection or an abnormality in the sympathetic nervous system.

Clinical features

- Hemifacial atrophy is characterized by gradual wasting of one side of the face and forehead.
- This usually starts between 5 years of age and the late teens.
- The wasting typically continues for a number of years before gradually stopping.
- The patient is then left with a permanent soft-tissue deficiency on one side of the face.
- The following sites are commonly affected:
  - The skin
    - Localized atrophy may occur.
  - The hair
    - Pigment changes or loss may be present.
  - The iris
    - Pigment changes may occur.
  - The forehead
    - A sharp depression, occasionally extending into the hairline, may be present.
    - This is known as 'coup de sabre'.
  - The cheek
    - The soft tissues of the cheek atrophy.
  - The skeleton
    - Underlying skeletal hypoplasia may be present.

Treatment

- Generally, no treatment is performed while the condition is active and progressive.
- Reconstruction is performed once the condition has been stable for at least 6 months. Reconstructive options include:
  1. Fat and dermofat grafts
  2. Temporoparietal fascia and temporalis muscle transfers

3 Free-tissue transfer
4 Osteotomies to correct the skeletal abnormalities.

- Free-tissue transfer is often performed in severe cases. Common transfers include:
  1 The scapular flap
  2 The parascapular flap
  3 The omentum.
- The defect should be slightly overcorrected to allow for subsequent flap atrophy.

Hyperplastic conditions

Fibrous dysplasia

- This condition is characterized by abnormal proliferation of bone forming mesenchyme.
- It occurs in the membranous bones of children.
- It usually presents as an enlarging mass in the maxilla or mandible.
- Lesions are usually osseous rather than fibrous.
- Cherubism is a condition also known as familial fibrous dysplasia.
  - It is characterized by multiple areas of fibrous dysplasia within the mandible and maxilla.
  - These lesions may occur as early as the 1st year of life.
- Albright's syndrome is characterized by the following.
  - Polyostotic fibrous dysplasia
  - Precocious puberty
  - Café-au-lait skin lesions
  - Tumours of the pituitary gland.

Treatment

- This consists of resection of the abnormal areas.
- The resultant defects are usually reconstructed with carved calvarial bone grafts.
- Radiotherapy may induce malignant transformation.

Cleft lip

Cleft lip

- CL is a congenital abnormality of the primary palate.
- The primary palate lies anterior to the incisive foramen and consists of:
  - The lip
  - The alveolus
  - The hard palate anterior to the incisive foramen.

Cleft palate

- CP is a congenital abnormality of the secondary palate.
- The secondary palate lies posterior to the incisive foramen and consists of:
  - The hard palate posterior to the incisive foramen.
  - The soft palate.

Cleft lip and cleft palate

- Both CL and CP may be:
  - Complete or incomplete
  - Unilateral or bilateral
    - Unilateral clefts of the palate occur when the vomer remains attached to one palatal shelf.
    - Bilateral clefts of the palate occur when the vomer is not attached to either palatal shelf.

Incidence

- In Caucasians, CL or CP occurs approximately once in 1000 live births.
- In Asia, the incidence is higher (once in 500 live births).
- In Africa, the incidence is lower (0.4 in 1000 live births).
- Combined CL&P is the most common deformity (45%).
- Isolated CP occurs in approximately 30% of cases.
- Isolated CL occurs in approximately 20% of cases.
- The ratio of left : right : bilateral CL is 6 : 3 : 1.

The aetiology of CL and CL&P differs in the following ways to that of isolated CP.

CL and CL&P

- Is twice as common in males.
- Has a familial association.
  - The relative risk of a child having CL or CL&P is:
    - No history of CL or CL&P in the family: 0.1%
    - One affected sibling: 4%
    - Two affected siblings: 9%.
    - One parent and one sibling affected: 17%
- CL and CL&P is infrequently associated with other abnormalities or syndromes.
  - Van der Woude syndrome is one of the few syndromes associated with CL.
  - It has the following characteristics:
    - Autosomal dominance
    - Multiple pits in the lips
    - Absence of second premolar teeth.

Isolated CP

- Is twice as common in females.
- Occurs in association with other abnormalities or as a part of a syndrome in up to 60% of cases.
- Is associated with environmental rather than familial factors.

Mechanism

- CL is thought to be caused by either:
  - Failure of fusion between the medial nasal process and the maxillary process; or

- Failure of mesenchymal penetration into the layer between the ectoderm and endoderm.
- This results in a breakdown between the processes after they have initially fused.

Anatomy

- Complete CL deformity is characterized by the following:
  1 Discontinuity in the skin and soft tissue of the upper lip.
  2 Vertical soft-tissue deficiency on the cleft side.
  3 Abnormal attachments of the lip musculature into the alar base and nasal spine.
  4 A cleft in the alveolus usually found at the site of subsequent canine tooth eruption.
  5 A defect in the hard palate anterior to the incisive foramen.
  6 Nasal deformity.
- A Simonart's band is a bridge of tissue lying across the upper lip.
- If this band occupies less than one-third of the vertical lip height, the resultant deformity is classified as a complete CL.
- If the band occupies more than one-third of the vertical lip height, the resultant deformity is classified as an incomplete CL.
- Forme fruste or microform clefts are a very mild form of incomplete CL.
- One or more of the following features may be present in a forme fruste:
  - A kink in the alar cartilage
  - A notch in the vermilion
  - A fibrous band across the lip.

Anatomy of the cleft nose deformity

The nasal anomaly associated with a CL is a complex three-dimensional deformity, which typically includes:

1 Deviation of the nasal spine, columella and caudal septum away from the cleft side.
2 Separation of the domes of the alar cartilages at the nasal tip.
3 Dislocation of the upper lateral nasal cartilage from the lower lateral cartilage on the cleft side.
4 A kink in the lateral crus of the lower lateral cartilage on the cleft side.
5 Retrodisplacement of the nasal base on the cleft side.
6 Flattening and displacement of the nasal bone on the cleft side.

Classification

- Kernahan has described a graphical classification of CL and CP.
- This classification likens the CL&P deformity to the letter 'Y'.
- Each anatomical area is allocated an area on the Y.
- Stippling of a box indicates a cleft in that area.
- Cross-hatching indicates a submucous cleft.
- Millard and Jackson have subsequently described modifications to Kernahan's original Y classification.

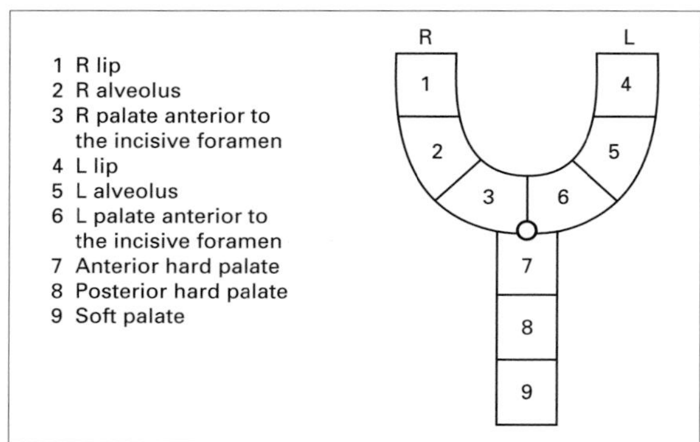

Timing of repair

- Cleft repair was traditionally performed when the child had attained the three '10's.
  1. Weight >10 lbs
  2. Age >10 weeks
  3. Haemoglobin >10 g/dl.
- Due to a relative lack of prospective randomized trials, there is little firm evidence as to the optimum timing of cleft repair.

Options include the following.

Repair in the neonatal period

- There is some debate as to how soon after birth surgery qualifies as neonatal.
- Generally surgery within 48 h of birth is classified as neonatal.
- Proponents of neonatal repair claim that it has the following advantages:
  - Better psychologically for both parent and child.
  - Better wound-healing with less inflammation and scarring.
- Disadvantages of neonatal repair include:
  - Difficulty in preoperative diagnosis of associated conditions, i.e. CVS abnormalities.
  - Technical difficulties due to the small size of the lip and palate.
  - The fact that neonates are obligate nasal breathers and can develop airway problems post-operatively.
  - Logistical problems in availability of surgeons and anaesthetists at short notice.
- Overall, there is little evidence that neonatal cleft repair confers a significant advantage.

Conventional repair

- The lip and anterior palate are repaired at approximately 3 months of age.
- The remaining cleft in the hard and soft palate is repaired at approximately 6 months of age.

Delaire technique

- The lip and soft palate are repaired between 6 and 9 months of age.
- The remainder of the palate is repaired between 12 and 18 months of age.
- This timing may result in better midfacial growth as less palatal dissection is required at the second operation.

Schweckendiek technique

- The lip and soft palate are repaired before the child is 1 year of age.
- The hard palate is repaired at approximately 8 years of age.
- Excellent midfacial growth is reported due to reduced disturbance of the important growth centres around the palate.
- Poor speech, due to palatal incompetence, has been reported in an independent audit.

Presurgical orthopaedics

- Presurgical orthopaedics involve the application of devices which:
  - Narrow the cleft deformity
  - Correct the alignment of the alveolar processes.
- Proponents claim this:
  - Makes subsequent surgical repair easier
  - Improves outcome.
- There are two main types of presurgical orthopaedic appliances.
  1. Passive appliances
     - These include obturators or feeding plates.
     - They prevent displacement of the alveolar arch by reducing the distorting forces produced by tongue movement.
  2. Dynamic appliances
     - These include the Latham appliance.
     - This is fixed to the maxilla and exerts an active force on the cleft deformity.
- Not all units utilize presurgical orthopaedics and their use is controversial.
- Some reserve their use for severe deformities such as a wide bilateral cleft of the lip and palate.
- There is some evidence that presurgical orthopaedics may be detrimental to subsequent growth.

Techniques of repair

- Many techniques of CL repair have been described.
- Each includes a method of lengthening the shortened lip on the cleft side.
- Whichever technique is used, it is important to:
  - Detach the abnormal muscle insertions
  - Reconstruct the lip musculature.
- Methods of CL repair can be categorized into the following:
  - **Straight-line techniques**
    - Rose–Thompson
    - Mirault–Blair–Brown–McDowell.
  - **Upper-lip Z-plasties**
    - Millard
    - Wynn.
  - **Lower-lip Z-plasties**
    - Tennison–Randall
    - Le Mesurier.

- **Upper- and lower-lip Z-plasties**
  - Skoog
  - Trauner.
- Among the most commonly used techniques are those described by Millard and Tennison–Randall.

The Millard rotation advancement technique

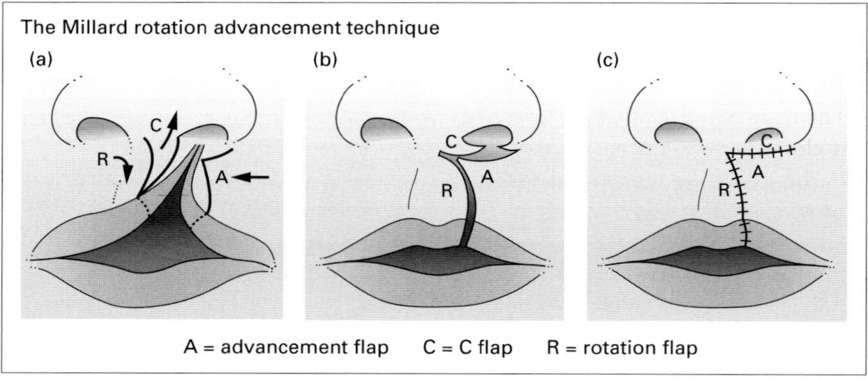

- Advantages:
  - The scar is located along, and disguised by, the philtral columns.
  - It is possible to adjust the degree of lip lengthening during surgery, hence it has been labelled a 'cut-as-you-go technique'.
  - Secondary revision is possible by re-elevation and rerotation of the flaps.
- Disadvantages:
  - It is a difficult technique to learn.
  - It places a scar across the philtrum at the nasal base.

The Tennison–Randall technique

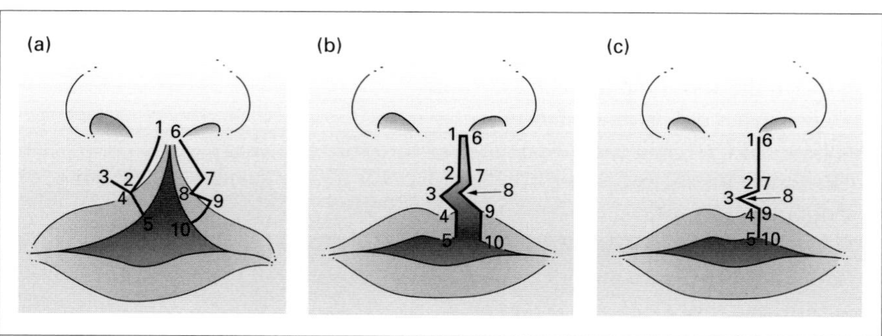

- This technique was originally described by Tennison, the geometry was further elucidated by Randall.

- Advantages:
  - The technique is relatively easy to learn.
- Disadvantages:
  - It is not easy to adjust the degree of lip lengthening intra-operatively.
  - The scar crosses the lower aspect of the philtral column.

Primary nasal surgery

- Correction of the nasal deformity associated with CL may be performed primarily at the time of lip repair, or delayed until nasal growth is complete.
- Delayed correction is usually performed in the late teenage years via an open rhinoplasty approach.
- The nasal deformity will be improved to some extent by repositioning the facial muscles into their normal locations during primary CL repair.

The following techniques can be used to correct the nasal deformity at the time of CL repair.

McComb technique

- This involves dissection over the dorsum of the nose in the plane between the nasal cartilages and the skin.
- Percutaneous sutures are then placed through the mobilized nasal cartilages to hold them in position.

Tajima technique

- An intranasal, reversed U-incision is used to access the alar cartilages.
- A trapezoidal suture is then placed between the cartilages to correct the nasal deformity.

Matsuma splints

- This technique utilizes nasal splints to mould the nasal cartilages.
- The splints are available in a number of sizes and are placed into the nostril.
- The pressure that they exert on the lower-lateral cartilages is believed to reduce the nasal deformity.

Alveolar bone grafting

- Alveolar bone grafting involves insertion of bone graft into the alveolar gap at the site of the cleft.
- It is usually performed at about the time when the permanent canine is about to erupt into the cleft.
- This normally occurs between 8 and 12 years of age.
- It is performed at this time because the canine will not erupt correctly into a bony alveolar defect.
- Timing of canine eruption is assessed by:
  - Observing when the contralateral upper canine is about to erupt.
  - X-ray examination.

3

- Alveolar bone grafting involves:
  - Harvesting cancellous bone graft from the iliac crest.
  - Packing the graft into the alveolar defect.
  - Covering the graft with local gingivoperiosteal flaps.
- Primary bone grafting at the time of the lip repair is performed in some centres.
- This is controversial as:
  - The bone may reabsorb.
  - Securing the dental arch at an early age may have a detrimental effect on facial growth.
- Primary mucoperiosteal flap closure of the alveolus can be performed at the time of the lip repair.
- This too is controversial as it makes subsequent bone grafting difficult and may hinder facial growth.

Bilateral cleft lip

- This defect is characterized by bilateral defects in the lip, alveolus and anterior palate.
- The central segment of the lip is the remnant of the medial nasal process of the frontonasal prominence, and consists of a:
  - Soft-tissue element called the prolabium
  - Skeletal element called the premaxilla.
- Initially, the premaxilla is often protuberant as its growth is unrestrained.
- However, as the child grows, it becomes relatively hypoplastic.
- Many of the early techniques to correct bilateral CL deformities involved removal of the premaxilla.
- These operations resulted in severe deformities of the upper lip and nose.
- Other techniques involved fracturing the vomer and setting the premaxilla back.
- These had a detrimental effect on facial growth as they disrupted important growth areas centered around the anterior nasal spine.

Techniques

- Presurgical orthopaedics with a Latham appliance, bonnets, bands or steristrips may narrow the cleft prior to surgery.
- Lip adhesion prior to definitive repair may be performed; this involves suturing the lip elements together to narrow the cleft.
- Staged surgery to one side before the other may be necessary in very wide cleft deformities.
- Many techniques have been used to correct the bilateral CL deformity. Among the most commonly used are:
  - **The Millard repair**
    - This technique is often used if the prolabium is relatively large.
    - The prolabium is raised off the underlying premaxilla.
    - Superiorly raised, forked flaps are then created from the lateral part of the prolabium.
    - These flaps are then turned laterally to run under the alar bases.

- The muscle bundles from the lateral lip elements are then isolated and sutured to each other across the midline.
- The central part of the prolabium is then replaced over the muscle to reconstruct the philtrum.

- **The Manchester repair**
  - This technique is often used when the prolabium is relatively small.
  - A longitudinal straight-line incision is made down either side of prolabium.
  - The prolabium is then sutured to the lateral lip elements in layers.

Cleft palate

Embryology

- Palatal development occurs between the 7th and 10th weeks of intra-uterine life.
- The lip is formed earlier, between the 4th and 8th weeks.
- The palatal shelves of the maxilla are initially orientated vertically.
- As the head grows and the neck straightens, the tongue falls away allowing the palatal shelves to rotate upwards into their normal horizontal position.
- Movement of the palatal shelves is thought to be an active process mediated by growth factors and hyaluronic acid.
- If the tongue does not descend adequately, it blocks upward rotation of the palatal shelves.
- This may result in a palatal cleft.

Anatomy of the palate

- CP is an abnormality in the secondary palate.
- The secondary palate lies posterior to the incisive foramen and is made up of the hard palate anteriorly and the soft palate posteriorly.
- The hard palate is composed of:
  - The palatal processes of the maxilla anteriorly
  - The palatine bones posteriorly.
- The soft palate contains the following muscles:
  - Tensor veli palatini
    - This muscle originates around the Eustachian tube.
    - It passes around the hamular process of the pterygoid plate and inserts into the palatine aponeurosis.
  - Levator veli palatini
    - This muscle originates around the Eustachian tube.
    - It descends downwards to insert from above and behind into the palatine aponeurosis.
    - It is the main functional muscle of the soft palate.
    - It elevates the soft palate and closes the opening between the nasopharynx and oropharynx.
  - Muscularis uvulae
    - This relatively small muscle lies within the uvula at the centre of the palate.

- It may be small or absent in submucous CP.
- The greater palatine vessels are the predominant vascular supply to the palate.

· These pass anteriorly and medially from the greater palatine foramen, situated at the posteriolateral border of the palate.

Anatomy of the cleft palate

- If the cleft involves the full length of the secondary palate, it is termed 'complete'.
- Incomplete clefts involve a segment of the secondary palate.
- CP may be unilateral or bilateral.
- Unilateral CP occurs if the vomer is attached to one palatal shelf.
- Bilateral CP occurs if the vomer is not attached to either palatal shelf.
- An occult submucous CP occurs when the palate looks normal but functions abnormally.

Environmental causes

- CP, as opposed to CL and CL&P, may be associated with the following:
  - Fetal alcohol syndrome
  - Anticonvulsant use
  - Maternal diabetes
  - Retinoic acid anomalies.
- There is some evidence that maternal folate supplements may reduce the incidence of CP.

Associated syndromes

- CP, as opposed to CL and CL&P, is commonly associated with other abnormalities and often occurs as part of a syndrome.
- Syndromes associated with CP include:
  - Velocardiofacial (VCF) syndrome
  - Treacher Collins syndrome
  - Stickler's syndrome
  - Apert's syndrome
  - Crouzon's syndrome
  - Down's syndrome.
- Pierre Robin sequence is termed a sequence rather than a syndrome as one event, a small jaw, results in:
  1. Limited tongue descent.
  2. This in turn prevents upward rotation of the palatal shelves.
  3. The paired palatal shelves do not fuse in the normal fashion and a wide, U-shaped CP results.

Velocardiofacial syndrome

- VCF syndrome is also known as:
  - DiGeorge syndrome
  - CATCH 22 syndrome
    - **C**: cardiac anomalies

- **A**: abnormal face
- **T**: thymic aplasia
- **C**: cleft palate
- **H**: hypocalcaemia
- **22**: the genetic abnormality is on the long arm of chromosome 22 (22q11 deformity).

- Characteristic facial features of this syndrome include:
  - A long face that is flat both physically and in expression
  - Epicanthic folds
  - A pinched nasal tip.
- Approximately 25% of affected individuals have abnormally positioned carotid arteries.
- These are often deviated towards the midline making surgery to the posterior pharyngeal wall hazardous.
- 10% of affected patients develop psychological problems in later life.
- This has elicited considerable interest as it is one of the few known genetic abnormalities associated with psychological illness.

Surgical repair of CP

Hard palate

- A number of techniques of CP repair have been described.
- In general, the palate is repaired in two layers.
- The nasal mucosa, on the upper surface of the palate, is repaired by suturing the mucosa on the nasal surface of the palate to that of the vomer.
- The following techniques are used to close the oral surface of the palate.

Veau–Kilner–Wardill technique

- This technique is also known as 'the push back'.
- Triangular mucoperiosteal flaps, with their apex sited anteriorly, are raised from either side of the oral surface of the palate.
- Each flap is based posteriorly on the greater palatine vessels.
- The oral layer of the cleft is repaired by suturing the mobilized flaps to each other along the midline.
- Following repair, there is no bony continuity across the cleft.
- New bone is formed by the periosteum within the flaps and bony continuity across the cleft is established.

Von Langenbeck technique

- Longitudinal incisions are made through the mucoperiosteum along the inner aspect of each alveolar arch.
- The incisions extend backwards from the level of the canine teeth to the level of the posterior limit of the alveolar arch.
- Bipedicled flaps are created by elevating the mucoperiosteum between the incisions laterally and the border of the cleft medially.

- The flaps are then transposed medially and sutured together in the midline.
- Each flap receives its blood supply from the greater palatine vessels.
- This technique, unlike 'the push back', avoids an incision in the anterior portion of the palate.
- This area is believed to contain important maxillary growth centres.
- Reduced dissection in this site may reduce subsequent facial undergrowth.

Medial von Langenbeck technique

- This is similar to the conventional von Langenbeck repair except that the releasing incisions are based more medially.
- The bipedicled flaps are therefore not as wide as in the conventional repair.
- Reduced lateral dissection may improve subsequent palatal growth.

Simple repair with no flaps

- In some narrow clefts, it may be possible to elevate mucoperiosteal flaps along the borders of the cleft and suture them together without the need for lateral releasing incisions.
- The reduced dissection may improve subsequent palatal growth.
- In order to reduce the width of the cleft and facilitate simple repair, some authors have advocated repairing the soft palate at the time of lip repair.
- The constraining forces of the musculature of the lip anteriorly and the soft palate posteriorly narrow the width of the palatal cleft and facilitate simple repair.

Soft palate

- When repairing the soft palate, it is important to detach abnormal muscle insertions into the back of the hard palate and reconstruct the normal muscular sling.
- The following techniques are commonly used to repair clefts in the soft palate.

Intravelar veloplasty

- The edges of the cleft are incised and the muscles of the soft palate are released from the posterior edge of the hard palate and the oral and nasal mucosa.
- The palate is then repaired in three layers:
  1. The nasal mucosa
  2. The muscle
  3. The oral mucosa.
- The lateral extent of the muscle dissection is variable.
- Some authors advocate dissection as far laterally as the pterygoid hamulus.

Furlow technique

- This technique involves lengthening the palate with two opposing Z-plasties.
- The first Z-plasty is based on the mucosa on the nasal surface of the soft palate.
- The second is designed in the opposite direction and is based on the mucosa of the oral surface of the soft palate.
- The intervening muscle layer is included in the posteriorly based flap of each Z-plasty.

- The muscle sling is reconstructed by suturing the muscle bundles contained in the posteriorly based flaps to one another.

Velopharyngeal incompetence

- During articulation movement of the soft palate and the pharyngeal walls controls air entry into the nasopharanx.
- Velopharygeal incompetence (VI) results from inability to fully close the space between the soft palate and the anterior wall of the pharynx.
- The sounds M, N and NG are nasal consonants, articulation of which requires air passage from the oropharynx into the nasopharanx.
- Articulation of the plosives B and P and the fricatives F and S require closure of the velopharangeal orifice.
- If the soft palate is incapable of closing the velopharangeal orifice, air escapes into the nose, resulting in characteristic hypernasal speech.
- Velopharyngeal closure is assessed by the following techniques:
  - **Video fluoroscopy**
    - This is a lateral soft-tissue x-ray.
    - Movement of the soft palate and pharynx is screened in real time.
    - Upward movement of the soft palate towards the posterior wall of the pharynx can be assessed.
  - **Nasoendoscopy**
    - A flexible endoscope is inserted through the nose to lie just above the velopharangeal orifice.
    - The pattern and degree of velopharyngeal closure can be visualized.
    - The method of pharyngoplasty is tailored to the pattern of velopharyngeal closure.

Pharyngoplasty

- This is an operation performed on the pharyngeal wall which aims to improve the closure of the velopharyngeal orifice.
- Techniques of pharyngoplasty can be divided into those based on its posterior wall and those based on its lateral wall.

Posterior wall pharyngoplasties

Operations based on the posterior wall include:

- **Pharyngeal wall augmentation**
  - Historically, Teflon, silicone and cartilage have been used to augment the pharyngeal wall.
- **Superiorly based pharyngeal flap elevation**
  - In this procedure, a superiorly based flap is elevated from the pharyngeal wall and inset into the soft palate.
  - Passage of air from the oro- into the nasopharynx occurs either side of the flap.
  - The superiorly based flap is usually preferred to the alternate inferiorly based design because:
    - As it contracts, its pull is upwards.
    - Theoretically its nerve supply, which enters from above, is preserved.

- **Inferiorly based flap**
  - In this procedure, an inferiorly based flap is elevated from the pharyngeal wall and inset into the soft palate.

Lateral wall pharyngoplasties

Operations based on the lateral wall include:

- **Hynes pharyngoplasty**
  - Two superiorly based flaps are raised from either side of the pharyngeal wall.
  - Each flap is 3–4 cm long and includes a portion of the salpingopharyngeus muscle and its overlying mucosa.
  - The flaps are then transposed medially and sutured to each other on the posterior pharyngeal wall.
- **Orticochoea pharyngoplasty**
  - Flaps are raised from the posterior tonsillar pillars.
  - Each flap contains a portion of the underlying palatopharyngeus muscle.
  - The flaps are transposed medially and interdigitated on the posterior pharyngeal wall.
  - The flaps are not sutured to the posterior pharyngeal wall laterally.
- **Jackson's modification of the Orticochoea pharyngoplasty**
  - This technique is similar to that described by Orticochoea.
  - It differs in the following ways:
    - The flaps are based higher.
    - The tips of the flaps are sutured end-to-end rather than interdigitated.
    - No lateral ports are left unsutured.

Complications following pharyngoplasty

- Respiratory obstruction
- Obstructive sleep apnoea
- Snoring.

Head and neck cancer

TNM classification

- When discussing head and neck cancer, it is important to be familiar with the TNM classification.
- The N and M classifications are universal for most tumours of the head and neck.
- T staging differs between tumours.

N and M classification for head and neck tumours

- Nx: the regional nodes cannot be assessed.
- N0: no regional lymph node metastases.
- N1: a single ipsilateral lymph node <3 cm in diameter.
- N2a: a single ipsilateral lymph node 3–6 cm in diameter.
- N2b: multiple ipsilateral lymph nodes not >6 cm in diameter.
- N2c: bilateral or contralateral lymph nodes 3–6 cm in diameter.

- N3: a lymph node >6 cm in diameter.
- Mx: the presence of metastases cannot be assessed.
- M0: no distant metastases.
- M1: distant metastases.

T classification of salivary gland tumours

- The T classification of salivary gland tumours is similar to that of the oral cavity except that each category is subdivided into 'a' and 'b'.
  - 'a' signifies no local extension of the tumour.
  - 'b' signifies local extension of the tumour into skin, soft tissue, muscle, bone or nerve.
- A T2a tumour, for example, is a tumour 2–4 cm in diameter which does not have any local extension.
  - Microscopic extension alone is not classified as local extension.

	Oral cavity and oropharyngeal tumours	Nasopharyngeal tumours	Hypopharyngeal tumours	Maxillary sinus tumours
T1	Primary tumour <2 cm diameter	Confined to one subsite	Confined to one subsite	Limited to the antral mucosa
T2	Primary tumour 2–4 cm diameter	In more than one subsite	In more than one subsite with no fixation	Invades the bone below the Ohngren's line
T3	Primary tumour >4 cm diameter	Extends beyond the nasal cavity	Invades the larynx	Invades the bone above the Ohngren's line
T4	Primary tumour invades adjacent structure	Invades the skull base or cranial nerves	Invades the soft tissues of the neck	Invades the adjacent structures

Staging of head and neck cancer

Stage 1	T1	N0	M0
Stage 2	T2	N0	M0
Stage 3	T3	N0	M0
	T0	N1	M0
	T1	N1	M0
	T2	N1	M0
	T3	N1	M0
Stage 4	T4	N0 or 1	M0
	Any T	N2 or 3	M0
	Any T	Any 0	M1

Levels of the neck

The neck has been subdivided into the following five levels.

Level 1: the submandibular triangle

This level lies below the inferior border of the mandible and above both bellies of the digastric muscle.

Level 2: the upper jugular region

- This level extends horizontally from the lateral border of sternohyoid muscle to the posterior border of the sternocleidomastoid muscle.
- Level 2 extends downwards from the skull base to the bifurcation of the carotid artery.
- The hyoid bone is the clinical landmark of the lower border.
- This level contains the upper jugular and jugulodigastric lymph nodes.

Level 3: the middle jugular region

- Its anterior and posterior borders are similar to those of level 2.
- Level 4 extends downwards from the bifurcation of the carotid artery to the omohyoid muscle.
- The cricothyroid membrane is the clinical landmark of the lower border.
- This level contains the middle jugular lymph nodes.

Level 4: the lower jugular region

- The anterior and posterior borders of this level are similar to those of levels 2 and 3.
- Vertically, level 4 extends downwards from the omohyoid to the clavicle.
- This level contains the lower jugular lymph nodes and the thoracic duct on the left side.

Level 5: the posterior triangle

- The anterior border of level 5 is the posterior edge of the sternocleidomastoid muscle.
- The posterior border is the anterior edge of trapezius, and the inferior border is the clavicle.
- This region contains branches of the cervical plexus and the transverse cervical artery.

Neck dissection

The nomenclature of neck dissection can be confusing. A neck dissection may be:

- Comprehensive: aims to remove the contents of all five levels of the neck.
- Selective: aims to remove the contents of some, but not all, of the levels.

Comprehensive neck dissection

Radical

In addition to removing the contents of all five levels of the neck, the following structures are removed:

- The internal jugular vein (IJV)
- The sternocleidomastoid muscle
- The accessory nerve.

Modified radical

- In recent years, there has been a move away from radical neck dissection in an effort to preserve functional structures whenever oncologically safe to do so.
- Modified radical neck dissection has been classified into the following three types:
  - *Type 1*: the accessory nerve is preserved.
  - *Type 2*: the accessory nerve and the sternocleidomastoid muscle are preserved.
  - *Type 3*: the accessory nerve, sternocleidomastoid muscle and the IJV are preserved.
- Functional neck dissection is a type of modified radical neck dissection.
- In order to avoid confusion, it is probably better to avoid the term 'functional neck dissection'.

Extended radical

In addition to removing the contents of all five levels of the neck, the dissection can be extended to include:

- Paratracheal nodes
- Mediastinal nodes
- The parotid gland.

Selective neck dissection

- Each tumour has a characteristic pattern of spread.
- It is therefore possible to selectively clear the levels most likely to be involved.
- This avoids unnecessary morbidity associated with removing tissue from neck levels which are unlikely to be involved.
- Clearing the tissue from some, but not all, of the levels in the neck is known as selective neck dissection.

The following are examples of selective neck dissection.

Supraomohyoid

- The contents of levels 1, 2 and 3 are removed in this procedure.
- It is often indicated in patients with oral cavity tumours, as these lesions preferentially drain into these levels.
- The risk of damaging the thoracic duct, which lies in level 4, is reduced in this procedure.

Anterolateral
· The contents of levels 2, 3 and 4 are removed in this procedure.
· It is often indicated in patients with laryngeal and hypopharyngeal tumours as these lesions preferentially drain to these levels.

Anterior
· The contents of levels 2, 3 and 4, plus the tracheo-oesophageal nodes, are removed in this procedure.
· It is often indicated in patients with thyroid tumours, as these lesions preferentially drain to these levels.

Posterior
· The contents of levels 2, 3, 4 and 5 are removed in this procedure.
· It is often indicated in patients with tumours in the posterior scalp, as these lesions preferentially drain to these levels.

Indications
- There is considerable debate as to the indications for neck dissection.
- As a general guide, radical neck dissections are usually performed on:
  - Patients with high-grade tumours with a clinically N2 neck.
  - Patients with recurrent disease.
  - Patients with invasive nodal disease i.e. involving the accessory nerve high in the neck.
- Modified radical neck or selective neck dissections are indicated for:
  - T3, T4 and N1 tumours.
  - T2 tumours of tongue.
  - If access is required to expose the neck vessels for microsurgical flap transfer.
  - In patients with high-risk tumours in whom adequate follow-up aimed at detecting neck involvement is impossible.
  - In patients with high-risk tumours with thick necks in whom detection of subsequent nodal metastases may be difficult.
- These are general guidelines only and the decision as to whether to perform a neck dissection, and if so the type and extent of the surgery, should be judged on an individual basis.
- Indications for radiotherapy following neck dissection are also contentious:
  - Some authorities recommend that any patient with positive histology from a neck dissection receives radiotherapy.
  - Some reserve post-operative radiotherapy for those patients with N2 disease.
  - Most agree that extracapsular spread is an indication for post-operative radiotherapy.

Complications
- As in all operations, complications can be divided into:
  - Intra-operative
  - Early
  - Late.

- Of these, the complications may be:
  - Specific to the operation
  - General complications of anaesthesia and major surgery.

Specific early intra-operative

These include:

- Bleeding
- Air embolus
- Pneumothorax
- Carotid artery injury
- Injury to any of the following nerves—phrenic, vagus, brachial plexus, lingual, hypoglossal and glossopharyngeal.

Specific intermediate

These include:

- Skin-flap necrosis
- Carotid blow out
  - This is often fatal and tends to occur in patients with salivary fistulas or those who have undergone radiotherapy.
- Chyle leak
  - This occurs as a result of damage to the thoracic duct.
  - It normally presents with milky drainage from the neck or as a collection.
  - The volume of the leak can be reduced by instituting a fat-free diet.
  - If the leak is large, total parental nutrition (TPN) usually results in significant reduction in its volume.

Specific late

- Scar contracture
- Neuroma formation
  - These usually originate from the cut ends of the cervical plexus.
- Shoulder pain syndrome
  - The incidence of this syndrome is reduced if the accessory nerve is preserved.
- Cellulitis and facial oedema

Management of intra-operative bleeding from the upper end of the IJV

This is a common exam question.

- Tell the anaesthetist you have a bleeding problem.
- Prevent air embolus by controlling the vein distally.
- Try to isolate the bleeding point by:
  - Suction
  - Dissection of the surrounding tissues.
- If possible, repair or oversew the defect in the IJV.
- If this is not possible, plug the defect with a finger or gauze.
- Ask your assistant to apply pressure to the area while you finish the neck dissection.
- If the area continues to bleed, plug it with a segment of the sternocleidomastoid muscle.

Management of isolated metastatic cervical lymph nodes with an unknown primary

- This is a popular exam question and not an uncommon clinical scenario.
- Interestingly, prognosis is better than cases in which the primary is identified.
- The following points are important in managing this condition.

History

- General symptoms
  - i.e. Weight loss
  - Presence of night sweats suggests lymphoma.
- Local symptoms
  - Pain, ulceration and trismus may indicate the likely site of the primary lesion.

Examination

- General examination
  - It is important to look for evidence of cachexia and for the presence of secondaries.
- Local examination
  - Intra-oral examination should be performed with the aid of a head lamp.

Investigations

Biopsy of the node

- A sample of the node should be submitted for histological examination.
- This specimen is usually obtained by fine needle aspiration (FNA).
- If the FNA is negative, open biopsy should be considered.
- The incision for an open biopsy should lie along that of any subsequent neck dissection.

Chest x-ray

Hilar nodes are suggestive of lymphoma.

MRI or CT scan

These investigations image the neck and may suggest the site of the primary tumour.

Panendoscopy

- Panendsoscopy should be performed in an effort to locate the primary tumour and detect any synchronous lesions.
- The following areas should be visualized:
  - Nasopharynx
  - Oropharynx
  - Hypopharynx
  - Oesophagus
  - Stomach

- Larynx
- Trachea and upper bronchi.

Biopsy

- During the panendoscopy, biopsies should be taken from any abnormal areas.
- Additional biopsies should be taken from areas in which the primary is most likely to originate, which include:
  - Pyriform fossa
  - Nasopharnx
  - Tonsillar fossa
  - Base of the tongue.

Treatment

- On histological confirmation of metastatic lymph node involvement, a neck dissection should be performed.
- Post-operatively, if the location of the primary tumour has not been identified, radiotherapy should be directed to:
  - The likely primary sites
  - The neck.

Radiology

MRI

- In this procedure, tissue is excited by a high-powered magnet.
- On switching off the magnetic field, excited photons emit a radiofrequency wave.
- T1-weighted images show fat as white.
- T2-weighted images show water as white.
- Stir films are modified T2 images with the fat signal suppressed.
- T2 images are good for demonstrating inflammation as these areas have a high water content.

CT

- CT images can be differentiated from MRI images as the bone appears white in the former and dark in the latter.
- Scout films show the level and spacing of the cuts.
- Bone-weighted scans are darker and demonstrate bony architecture.
- Non-bone weighted scans are lighter and demonstrate soft tissues.
- Lymph nodes are significant if >1 cm in diameter.
- Malignant nodes on CT have a radiolucent core and a radio-opaque periphery.
- Lesions in the superficial lobe of the parotid lie lateral to the retromandibular vein.
- Lesions in the deep lobe of the parotid lie medial to the retromandibular vein and abut the internal carotid artery and the tonsillar region of the oropharynx.

Salivary gland tumours

- Salivary gland tumours account for approximately 3% of all head and neck malignancies.
- 80% occur in the parotid gland.
- 80% of parotid masses are benign.
- 50% of submandibular tumours are benign.

Factors suggestive of malignancy

The following factors suggest that a mass may be malignant:

- Pain
- Obstruction or infection
- Nerve involvement
- Invasion of other structures
- Bleeding from the duct
- Rapid progression.

Benign parotid tumours

These lesions are common and include the following.

Pleomorphic adenoma

- This tumour is also known as a benign mixed tumour.
- It is the commonest benign tumour of the parotid gland and usually presents as a slowly growing mass.
- Invasion of the facial nerve producing facial nerve palsy is extremely rare.
- Although seemingly well encapsulated, simple enucleation is associated with a high rate of local recurrence.
- Treatment is usually via superficial parotidectomy.

Adenolymphoma

- This tumour is also known as Warthin's tumour.
- It is classically located in the tail of the parotid gland in elderly males.
- 5–10% of tumours are bilateral.
- Most cases are treated by superficial parotidectomy.

Other benign tumours of the parotid gland

- Oncocytomas
- Sebaceous adenomas
- Cystadenomas

Malignant parotid tumours

- Most malignant parotid tumours arise within the body of the gland.
- They occasionally occur in the tail and rarely in the deep lobe.
- Malignant parotid lesions are either:
  - Primary parotid tumours, or
  - Secondary tumours, most of which originate from scalp or ear malignancies.

Primary tumours originating from the parotid gland include the following.

Mucoepidermoid carcinoma
· This lesion accounts for 30% of malignant parotid tumours.
· The tumour has three histological grades:
 1 Well-differentiated tumours which display limited local invasiveness and rarely metastasize.
 2 Intermediate-grade tumours which behave in a similar fashion to well-differentiated SCCs.
 3 Poorly differentiated tumours which behave as high-grade malignancies and are prone to local invasion and regional spread.

Adenoid cystic carcinoma
· This lesion accounts for approximately 20% of malignant parotid tumours.
· The tumour has three histological grades:
 1 The cibrose form has the best prognosis.
 2 The tubular form has an intermediate prognosis.
 3 The solid form has the worst prognosis.
· Skip lesions along the facial nerve are common and the tumour is particularly prone to perineural invasion.
· This tumour is notable for its ability to recur many years after its initial presentation, sometimes as lung metastases.
· There is some debate about whether patients with adenocytic carcinoma are ever cured.
· Some authorities believe that if patients are followed up for long enough, all develop recurrence.

Carcinoma ex pleomorphic adenoma
· This tumour arises from a pleomorphic adenoma.
· Malignant transformation usually occurs after a pleomorphic adenoma has been present for at least 10 years.

Other malignant tumours
· Adenocarcinoma
· Acinic cell tumour
· Sebaceous carcinoma
· Lymphoma.

Technique of superficial parotidectomy
Ideally, no muscle relaxant should be administered to facilitate identification of the facial nerve with a nerve stimulator.

Blair incision
· Commonly used, this incision starts at the upper anterior border of the ear, extends downwards along the preauricular crease and continues backwards over the mastoid process.
· From here it passes anteriorly in a cervical crease towards the hyoid bone.
· The neck incision lies approximately two finger breadths below the mandible.

Elevation of the skin flap
· The skin flap is elevated from the parotid gland.
· Care should be taken to preserve the greater auricular nerve as it may subsequently be required as a nerve graft.

Separation of the tail of the parotid gland
· The tail of the parotid gland is separated from the sternocleidomastoid and digastric muscles.
· Care must be taken not to damage the posterior facial vein as ligation causes venous congestion of the gland.

Approach to the facial nerve
· The facial nerve can be approached proximally as it enters the gland (antegrade approach) or distally as it exits the gland (retrograde approach).
· If the tumour is large, it may prove difficult to retract the parotid and a retrograde approach may be preferred.

The antegrade approach
· The cartilaginous tragal pointer should be visualized.
· The facial nerve can be found 1 cm deep to this point.
· A nerve stimulator can be used to confirm identification of the facial nerve.
· The superficial lobe of the parotid gland is then separated from the facial nerve by careful dissection along the perineural space.

The retrograde approach
The distal branches of the facial nerve can be identified at the following sites:
· The cervical branch as it runs alongside the retromandibular vein.
· The marginal branch below the lower border of the mandible as it runs superficially over the facial artery.
· The buccal branches as they run alongside the parotid duct (Stensen's duct). Identification of Stensen's duct may be aided by cannulation from inside the mouth.

Indications for post-operative radiotherapy
Post-operative radiotherapy should be considered for:
· Malignant parotid lesions
· Incompletely excised benign lesions.

Carcinoma of the lip
· The lip extends laterally to the nasolabial folds.
· Vertically, it extends from the base of the nose to the chin.
· The site at which the lip becomes the oral cavity lies at the junction of the wet and dry mucosa.
· The labial artery and vein course just beneath the mucosa on the lingual side of the lip.

- The commonest tumour affecting the lip is squamous cell carcinoma (SCC).
- This is usually associated with long-term sun exposure.
- Most tumours occur on the lower lip, possibly because it is exposed to more sunlight.
- Larger tumours and those arising from the mucosa are more likely to develop regional metastases.
- Tumours should be resected with a minimum margin of 5 mm.
- Large or poorly differentiated tumours require wider excision.
- Radiotherapy may be indicated for small tumours around the commissure as function may be difficult to restore after resection.

Reconstruction

- In 1920, Sir Harold Gillies stated the following principles of lip reconstruction: 'Restoration is designed from within outwards. The lining membrane must be considered first, then the supporting structures, and finally the covering.'
- Generally, defects that occupy less than 30% of the horizontal width of the lip can be reconstructed by direct closure.
- This is a general guideline and varies between individuals according to local tissue laxity.
- Lesions limited to the mucosa can be managed by excision of the vermilion and mucosal advancement.
- Reconstruction techniques for full-thickness defects occupying between 30% and 50% of the horizontal length of the lip include:
  - Johanson's step technique
  - Karapandzic flap reconstruction
  - Abbé flap reconstruction
  - Estlander flap reconstruction.
- Reconstruction techniques for full-thickness defects occupying over 50% of the horizontal length of the lip include:
  - Webster's modification of the Bernard lip reconstruction
  - Gillies' fan flap reconstruction
  - McGregor flap reconstruction.
- Details of these methods of reconstruction are beyond the scope of this book and readers are referred to more specialized texts.

Tumours of the oral cavity

Anatomy

- The oral cavity extents anteriorly to the wet–dry border of the lips.
- It extends posteriorly to the junction of the hard and soft palates above and the circumvallate papillae of the tongue below.
- The oral cavity contains:
  - The inner aspect of the lips
  - The buccal mucosa
  - The alveolar ridges

- The floor of the mouth
- The retromolar trigone
- The hard palate
- The anterior two-thirds of the tongue.

Aetiology and pathology

3

- Malignant tumours of the oral cavity account for approximately 30% of all head and neck malignancies.
- Of these, SCCs account for over 90% of primary carcinomas.
- Salivary gland tumours account for most of the other cases.
- Development of intra-oral carcinoma is associated with the six 'S's.
  1. **S**moking
  2. **S**pirits
  3. **S**pices
  4. **S**harp teeth
  5. **S**unlight
  6. **S**yphilis.
- Premalignant lesions include:
  - Leukoplakia
    - This presents as a white patch which, unlike lichen planus, cannot be scraped off.
    - Approximately 25–30% of untreated lesions undergo malignant transformation.
- Erythroplakia
    - This presents as a red patch.
    - *In situ* or invasive carcinoma is found in approximately 50% of these lesions.

Management

Important steps in managing intra-oral carcinoma include:

1. A full history
2. A detailed examination
    - It is important to assess the clinical TNM staging.
3. FNA of any neck masses
4. Chest x-ray
5. MRI or CT scan
    - These investigations are important to define the extent of the tumour.
    - It is particularly important to assess the extent of mandibular involvement.
    - These investigations may demonstrate clinically undetectable lymphatic involvement in the neck.
6. Pan-endoscopy
    - Pan-endoscopy should be performed on all patients with intra-oral malignancy as synchronous tumours will be found in 1–6% of patients.
    - Biopsies should be taken of any clinically suspicious areas.
    - Synchronous tumours occur within 6 months of the first tumour.
    - Metachronous tumours occur more than 6 months after the first tumour.

Treatment

- Many T1 or T2 tumours can be treated with brachytherapy (implant radiotherapy).
- Control rates are similar to surgery.
- Long-term function after brachytherapy is probably superior to surgery.
- Brachytherapy is probably not suitable for tumours abutting bone as osteoradionecrosis may result.
- Small T1 or T2 tumours can usually be accessed through the mouth.
- Adequate access to larger lesions may require a mandible splitting approach.
- Excision margins of 1–2 cm are recommended for most tumours.
- Approximately 40% of patients with tongue cancers have nodal involvement at the time of presentation; 20% of patients will have bilateral disease.
- It is generally agreed that therapeutic neck dissection should be performed on patients who have nodal involvement in the neck.
- Indications for prophylactic neck dissection are more contentious.
- Most units offer patients with T3 and T4 tumours elective node dissection.
- Patients with T1 tumours are unlikely to develop nodal metastases and elective neck dissection is not routinely performed.
- Some T2 tumours (particularly of the tongue) are prone to develop nodal disease.
- The decision as to whether to perform an elective neck dissection on patients with T2 tumours is therefore taken on an individual basis.

Reconstructive options

Reconstructive options following excision of intra-oral tumours include the following.

Direct closure

This may be suitable for small mobile lesions.

Skin grafts

- This method of reconstruction may be suitable for superficial defects on the tongue and palate.
- Due to graft contraction, this technique should probably not be used in sites such as the floor of the mouth where tethering and decreased mobility may result.

Local flaps

- Mucosal flaps, tongue flaps and palatal flaps can be used to reconstruct small defects.
- These flaps are less frequently used nowadays as improved techniques have been developed.

Regional flaps

The following regional flaps can be used to reconstruct intra-oral defects:

- Nasolabial flap
- Temporalis muscle and fascia flaps

- Forehead flap
- Deltopectoral flap
- Pectoralis major flap
- Latissimus dorsi flap
- Trapezius flap.

Free-tissue transfer

- The following free flaps are commonly used to reconstruct intra-oral defects:
  - Radial forearm flap (RFF)
  - Lateral arm flap
  - Rectus abdominis muscle flap
  - Jejunal flaps.
- Specific flaps are indicated for specific defects.
- Muscle-only flaps are often used to reconstruct the tongue after total glossectomy.
- Fascia-only flaps can be skin grafted and used to reconstruct thin defects such as those on the palate.
- Free-tissue transfer has the following advantages:
  - It offers greater flexibility in flap design and composition.
  - One-stage reconstruction is usually possible.
  - An element of sensation may be restored to the flap by neurotization.
  - It is associated with fewer complications in irradiated patients.

Mandibular reconstruction

- Mandibular periosteum is very resistant to tumour spread.
- Bone invasion can occur:
  1. Through the soft tissue (infiltrative spread)
  2. Along lymphatic channels (embolic spread)
  3. Along nerves (permeative spread)
  4. Through the occlusal surface following tooth extraction.
- Radiotherapy disrupts periosteal integrity causing it to lose its resistance to tumour spread.

Excision

Rim resection

- This involves resection of the alveolus with preservation of the body of the mandible.
- This technique is indicated in cases with only limited bony invasion.
- It should not be used after irradiation as this alters the pattern of tumour spread.

Segmental resection

- This type of resection is appropriate in cases with significant bony invasion, or those in which the mandible has been irradiated.

- Bony reconstruction is necessary after segmental excision.
- Segmental defects of the mandible are classified in the following way.
  - **C** is the central segment between the canine teeth.
  - **L** is the lateral segment not including the condyle.
  - **H** is the lateral segment including the condyle.
- Many defects are a combination of one of more segments.
  - LC, for example, is a segmental defect of the central and lateral mandible excluding the condyle.
  - LCL is a large central segmental defect sparing the condyles.

Reconstruction

No bone reconstruction

- Segmental bony defects can be spanned by contoured reconstruction plates.
- These are rigidly fixed to bone at either end of the defect.
- This form of reconstruction is best suited to patients who:
  1. Are not suited to other methods of reconstruction
  2. Have lateral defects
  3. Have good soft tissue coverage
  4. Have not received and will not receive radiotherapy.

Reconstruction with non-vascularized tissue

These techniques include:

- Non-vascularized, free-bone graft
- Freeze-dried, autoclaved or irradiated autogenous mandible
- Alloplastic materials such as titanium trays containing cancellous bone graft.

Vascularized tissue

- Vascularized bone is the optimal method of mandibular reconstruction.
- It has the advantage of being osseoinductive as well as osseoconductive (p. 30).
- Vascularized bone to reconstruct the mandible can be obtained from:
  - Pedicled transfer
  - Free-tissue transfer.
- Sources of vascularized bone for mandibular reconstruction by pedicled transfer include:
  - A segment of the clavicle pedicled on the sternocleidomastoid muscle
  - A segment of the scapula pedicled on the trapezius muscle
  - A segment of the rib or sternum pedicled on the pectoralis major muscle.

Sources of vascularized bone for mandibular reconstruction by free-tissue transfer include the following.

The deep circumflex iliac artery flap

- The deep circumflex iliac artery (DCIA) flap is suitable for hemimandibular reconstruction.
- The skin overlying the flap is relatively precarious.

· A segment of the internal oblique muscle, based on the ascending branch of the DCIA, may be included in the flap.

The radial-forearm flap

· The RFF has a good skin paddle but less than ideal bone.
· Up to 12 cm of bone is available in the adult between the insertions of pronator teres and brachioradialis.

The free-fibula flap

· This flap has the following advantages:
  · It is the longest vascularized bone available.
  · It has a dense cortical structure.
  · It is supplied by multiple perforators from the peroneal artery.
· This segmental supply permits the creation of multiple osteotomies to contour accurately the bone to the dimensions of the mandibular defect.
· While the free-fibula flap is an excellent source of bone, the skin paddle can be precarious.

The scapular flap

· This flap, based on the subscapular axis, can include a portion of the lateral border of the scapula.
· Up to 12–14 cm of bone is available.

Tumours of the nasal cavity and paranasal sinuses

· Tumours of the paranasal sinuses account for approximately 3% of head and neck malignancies.
· They are more common in the Far East.
· The following areas may be affected:
  1 The maxillary sinus
  2 The nasal cavity
  3 The ethmoid sinus
  4 The sphenoid sinus
  5 The frontal sinus.

Primary tumours

· Benign tumours
  · Osteomas
  · Fibromas
  · Fibrous dysplasia.
· Osseous malignant tumours
  · Osteogenic sarcoma
  · Ewing's sarcoma.
· Connective-tissue malignant tumours
  · Chondrosarcoma
  · Fibrosarcoma

  - Malignant fibrous histioctyoma (MFH)
  - Rhabdomyosarcoma.
- Epithelial tumours
  - SCC
  - Adenocarcinoma
  - Mucoepidermoid carcinoma
  - Malignant melanoma (MM).

Management
- The tumour should be staged with an MRI or CT scan.
- Biopsy should be performed to confirm the presence of a tumour.
- Tumours below Ohngren's line have a better prognosis.
- The maxillary sinus is usually approached via a Weber–Ferguson incision.
- The extent of the resection is tailored to the individual tumour.
- Total maxillectomy is less often performed now.
- The orbital floor is usually reconstructed with calvarial bone grafts.
- Maxillectomy defects can be lined with skin grafts.
- A dental plate can be used to recreate the function of the alveolus and palate.
- Reconstruction after maxillectomy can also be performed with DCIA or a rectus abdominis flap.

Facial fractures and soft-tissue injuries

General management principles

Important principles in the management of facial fractures include:
- Accurate diagnosis
- Early single-stage surgery
- Thorough exposure of all bony fragments
- Precise rigid fixation
- Immediate bone grafting where necessary
- Reconstruction and resuspension of the soft tissues.

Incisions for access

It may be possible to access the fracture through pre-existing lacerations. If no suitable lacerations exist, one or more of the following incisions will be required to expose the fracture.
- Bicoronal incision
- Lower-eyelid incision, at any of the following four sites:
  1. Through the conjunctiva (trans-conjunctival incision)
  2. Just below the eyelash margin (subciliary incision)
  3. Though the centre of the eyelid (mid-lid incision)
  4. At the junction of the eyelid and the cheek.
- Upper or lower buccal sulcus incision
- Dingman's lateral brow incision
- Risdon's retromandibular incision

- Lynch's medial canthus incision
- Gillies' incision within the hair-line of the temple.

Radiological investigation

The following radiological views are used to image fracture sites.

- Straight posteroanterior (PA) views
- Caldwell views
  - These are inclined PA views, taken with 23° of head extension.
- Waters' views
  - These are inclined PA views, taken with 37° of head extension.
- Towne's views
  - These are anteroposterior (AP) views, taken with the x-ray tube rotated 30° degrees in a caudal direction.
- Reverse Towne's views
  - These are similar to the conventional Towne's views except that the positions of the tube and plate are reversed.
- CT scan
- Three-dimensional CT reconstruction
  - This investigation may be useful in complex injuries but it does expose the patient to a significant dose of radiation.

Management of facial soft-tissue injuries

Skin

- Skin has a good blood supply and therefore usually only requires minimal debridement.
- Edges of lacerations should be excised before suturing.

Facial nerve

- Facial nerve branches medial to the lateral canthus are generally too small to repair.
- In most instances, the muscles will re-innervate spontaneously.
- Facial nerve branches are divided lateral to the outer canthus and should be repaired if possible.

Parotid duct

- The parotid duct (Stensen's duct) traverses the mid-third of the line drawn between the tragus and the corner of the mouth.
- The duct is closely related to buccal branches of the facial nerve.
- Duct injury should be suspected if there is any weakness in the muscles supplied by these branches.
- If doubt exists as to the integrity of the duct, a probe should be inserted into its intra-oral opening.

- This lies opposite the second upper premolar tooth.
- If the duct is divided, it should be repaired over a thin stent.
- Complications of not recognizing and repairing duct injuries include:
  - Salivary collections
  - Salivary fistulas
  - Stenosis of the duct
  - Parotitis.

Lacrimal apparatus

- Injuries to the canaliculi, lacrimal sac or lacrimal duct should be repaired over a fine silastic stent.
- The stent should be inserted along the length of the lacrimal system.
- Its ends are usually tied to each other externally to prevent it migrating.

Timing of surgery

- Management of other injuries, such as fractures of the cervical spine, take priority over the treatment of the facial fractures.
- Facial fracture fixation is performed as follows:
  - Early surgery
    - This is the preferred timing, provided that the patient is in a stable condition.
  - Delayed primary surgery
    - This is performed approximately 10 days following injury once facial swelling has settled.
    - Delayed primary surgery may be indicated in patients with multiple injuries.
  - Secondary surgery
    - Late surgery should generally be avoided as the soft tissues contract over the skeleton, making bony realignment difficult.

Immediate management of patients with pan-facial fractures

- This is a common question at all levels of exam.
- The patient should be examined in the order 'ABC':
  - **A**irway
  - **B**reathing
  - **C**irculation.

Airway

- The cervical spine should first be stabilized with a hard collar and sandbags.
- Any false or broken teeth should be removed.
- Vomitus and blood should be removed from the airway.
- If the patient is not maintaining their own airway:
  - The mandible should be distracted forward to provide tongue support.
  - The airway may be improved by reducing fractures by relocating the maxilla upwards and forwards.

- If the airway remains inadequate, it should be secured by one of the following means.
  - Intubation
  - Cricothyroidotomy
  - Tracheostomy.

Breathing

- Co-existing chest injury should be excluded.
- Ensure that the patient is adequately ventilated.

Circulation

- Insert large-bore cannulae and start an infusion.
- Send blood for haemoglobin estimation, glucose, urea and electrolytes, drug and alcohol screening and cross-matching.
- Profuse bleeding from facial fractures can be reduced by:
  - Manual reduction of the fractures
  - Nasal packing
- If bleeding is still profuse:
  1. Set up a blood transfusion and try to correct any coagulopathy.
  2. Administer suitable analgesia.
  3. Take the patient to the operating theatre.
- When the patient is anaesthetized:
  1. Try to reduce the fractures and hold them in place with temporary percutaneous K-wires.
  2. Consider facial bandaging
     - Facial bandaging consists of packing the mouth and nose and then applying circumferential facial bandages.
- If bleeding continues, consider external carotid artery ligation.
  - This can be performed:
    1. Through an incision behind the ramus of the mandible
    2. Endoscopically through the maxillary sinus.

Management of associated injuries

- Once the patient has been stabilized, it is important to exclude other injuries.
- 10% of patients with major facial fractures have cervical spine fractures.
- 10% of patients with major facial fractures have associated eye injuries.
- Ophthalmic assessment in patients with severe injuries is mandatory.

Mandibular fractures

Symptoms and signs

Mandibular fractures may present with the following signs and symptoms.

- Pain
- Trismus
  - This is difficulty in opening the mouth.

- Malocclusion
  - The patient may complain that their teeth do not fit together properly.
- Crepitus
- Bruising
  - This may be extra- or intra-oral.
- Palpation may reveal a step along the mandibular border or in the dentition.
- Paraesthesia may be present in the distribution of the inferior alveolar nerve.

Locations

Mandibular fractures occur as follows:

- Condyle: 36%
- Body: 20%
- Angle: 20%
- Symphysis: 14%
- Alveolus: 4%
- Ramus: 3%
- Coronoid process: 3%.

Common patterns

- Double fractures are common and tend to occur in the following combinations:
  1 The angle and the contralateral body.
  2 The parasymphysis and the contralateral subcondylar region.
  3 The symphysis and both condyles.
- If one fracture is present, it is important to exclude the presence of another.

Classification

- Fractures of the mandible may be closed or compound.
  - Fractures may be compound through:
    - The skin
    - The buccal mucosa
    - A tooth socket.
- Kazanjian and Converse have classified mandibular fractures in the following way:
  - *Class 1*: teeth on both bony fragments.
  - *Class 2*: teeth on one bony fragment.
  - *Class 3*: teeth on neither bony fragment.
- In addition, fractures may be classified as favourable or unfavourable.
- Unfavourable fractures:
  - Slope upwards and anteriorly from the lower border of the mandible.
  - Slope anteriorly and inwards in the transverse plane.
  - Are inherently unstable because of the pull of the following muscles:
    - Masseter
    - Digastric
    - The pterygoids.
  - The action of these muscles distracts the bony fragments at the fracture site.

- Fractures in the opposite direction are inherently stable as muscle action compresses the bony fragments at the fracture site.

Radiological investigation

- The following radiological investigations can be used to identify the site, extent and displacement of mandibular fractures:
  - An orthopantomogram (OPG)
  - A PA view
  - A lateral oblique view
  - A reverse Towne's view to visualize the condyles.
- CT scanning is usually of little additional value in isolated mandibular fractures.

Management

Conservative management

- This form of management is indicated for most condylar fractures (see below).
- It may also be used for stable, undisplaced fractures with normal occlusion.

Intermaxillary fixation

- In this technique, the teeth of the maxilla and mandible are wired together.
- IMF is so called because the mandible used to be known as the inferior maxilla.
- Fixation of the teeth of the mandible to those of the maxilla can be achieved by the application of:
  - Wires
  - Arch bars
  - Cap splints.
- These should not be attached to the incisors or canines as their single root makes them relatively unstable.
- IMF is usually maintained for 3–6 weeks.
- IMF does not provide rigid fracture fixation.
- Disadvantages of IMF include:
  - Difficulties in maintaining oral hygiene.
  - Eating difficulties which may lead to weight loss.
  - Potential airway obstruction.

Open reduction and internal fixation

- In recent years, open reduction and internal fixation (OR&IF) has become the preferred method of treating most mandibular fractures.
- Monocortical or bicortical fixation may be performed.
- Bicortical fixation risks damaging tooth roots.
- Champy's principle of tension band plating may be utilized.
- He noted that muscular forces on the mandible tend to distract its upper border and compress its lower border.
- Therefore, a plate on the upper border acts as a tension band producing compression at the lower border.

- This form of fixation is often used in fractures posterior to the mental foramen.
- Fractures anterior to the mental foramen are usually treated with upper and lower bicortical plate fixation.
- Internal fixation is performed via an intra-oral approach whenever possible.
- In difficult sites, a transcutaneous trocar passing through the cheek can be used to insert the screws.

External fixation

External fixation is rarely used nowadays but it may occasionally be indicated in patients with:

- Extensive bony defects
- Osteomyelitis.

Management of condylar fractures

- Treatment of condylar fractures is controversial.
- Intracapsular fractures are prone to ankylosis, particularly if immobilized.

Management options for condylar fractures include:

- Conservative management with a soft diet.
- Closed reduction and the application of IMF.
- OR&IF
  - OR&IF is indicated in the following cases:
    - When the condylar head is dislocated from the TMJ.
    - When the condyle is laterally displaced 30° or more from the axis of the ascending ramus.
    - In bilateral fractures associated with shortening of the ascending ramus and an anterior open bite.
    - If adequate occlusion cannot be achieved by closed reduction.
    - If there is a foreign body within the TMJ.

Zygomatic fractures

- The zygoma forms:
  1. The eminence of the cheek
  2. The inferolateral border of orbit.
- Zygomatic fractures tend to occur in a tetrapod fashion at its junction with:
  - The zygomatic process of the frontal bone at the zygomaticofrontal suture (ZF suture).
  - The greater wing of the sphenoid in the lateral orbit.
  - The maxilla in the orbital margin, orbital floor and anterior wall of the maxillary sinus.
  - The temporal bone in the zygomatic arch.

Symptoms and signs

Symptoms and signs of zygomatic fractures include:

- Bruising and swelling
  - These may be present over the zygoma and inside the mouth.

- Malar depression
- A palpable bony step
- Subconjunctival haematoma
  - This will have no posterior limit as the fracture line extends behind the orbital septum.
  - The haematoma is bright red due to transconjunctival oxygenation from the air.
- Trismus
  - This occurs when the zygomatic arch abuts the coronoid process of the mandible.
- Epistaxis
  - Epistaxis may be present due to a tear in the mucosal lining of the maxillary sinus.
- Paraesthesia in the distribution of the infra-orbital nerve
- Enophthalmos
  - This is posterior displacement of the globe of the eye.
  - Clinically, enophalmos can be detected by looking at the position of the globe from above the patient's head.
- Dystopia
  - This is alteration in the position of the orbit and its contents.
  - It is classified by the direction of orbital movement into:
    1 Lateral dystopia
    2 Vertical dystopia
    3 A combination of lateral and vertical dystopia.
- Diplopia
  - Diplopia is double vision.
  - It usually occurs on upward gaze due to trapping of the inferior rectus muscle.
  - Tethering of the orbital contents within fracture lines can be detected with the forced duction test.
  - In this test, the eye is first anaesthetized.
  - Gentle traction with forceps is applied to the inferior conjunctiva.
  - Limitation in globe movement indicates tethering of the orbital contents.
- Decreased visual acuity
  - This may be due to retinal detachment.
  - It is important to measure and record visual acuity in patients suspected of having fractures in the upper part of the face.

Radiological investigation

The following radiological investigations can be used to identify the site, extent and displacement of zygomatic fractures.

- PA views
- Lateral views
- Waters' views
  - These demonstrate the maxillary sinus.
- Caldwell views
  - These demonstrate the ZF suture.

- CT scanning
  - In complex injuries a three-dimensional reconstruction may be useful.

Classification

Zygomatic fractures have been classified by Knight and North into the following groups:

1 Undisplaced fractures: 6%
2 Isolated arch fractures: 10%
3 Unrotated body fractures: 33%
4 Zygomatic body fractures with medial rotation at the ZF suture: 11%
5 Zygomatic body fractures with lateral rotation at the ZF suture: 22%
6 Complex fractures: 18%.

Management

Zygomatic fractures can be managed in the following ways.

- Conservatively
  - Conservative treatment is usually reserved for stable undisplaced fractures.
- With a Gillies' lift
  - This procedure is indicated for displaced fractures of the zygomatic arch.
  - A Gillies' lift is performed in the following way:
    1 A radial incision is made above and anterior to the ear.
    2 The incision is deepened through the temporoparietal fascia (superficial temporal fascia).
    3 The deep temporal fascia lies deep to the temporoparietal fascia.
    4 The white deep temporal fascia is incised and a Gillies' elevator is inserted between it and the underlying temporalis muscle.
    5 This plane leads directly under the zygomatic arch.
    6 The fracture should be elevated by lifting.
    7 Pivoting the elevator on the temporal bone may result in secondary fracture.
- With OR&IF
  - In recent years, OR&IF has become the preferred method of treating many zygomatic fractures.
  - Plates should be placed over two or three of the fracture lines.
  - Fractures at the ZF suture are approached via a lateral brow incision.
  - Fractures in the infra-orbital rim are approached via a lower-eyelid incision.
  - Fractures in the maxilla are approached via an upper buccal sulcus incision.

Maxillary fractures

The maxilla is reinforced by three vertical and three horizontal buttresses.

- The vertical buttresses include the:
  1 Nasomaxillary buttress which lies along the junction of the cheek and the nose
  2 The zygomatico-maxillary buttress which passes through the body of the zygoma and upwards into the lateral orbital rim and zygomatic arch
  3 The pterygopalatine buttress which passes posteriorly.

- The horizontal buttresses pass through the:
  1 Infra-orbital rims
  2 The zygoma
  3 The alveolar arch.

Le Fort fractures

- René Le Fort was a French surgeon at the end of the 19th century.
- He observed the distribution of fractures in skulls dropped from upper-storey windows.
- He noted that fractures of the maxilla tend to occur in the following patterns.
- **Le Fort 1 fracture**
  - This is also known as a Geurin fracture.
  - The fracture line passes transversely across:
    1 The base of the piriform aperture
    2 The base of the maxillary sinus
    3 The pterygoid plates.
  - This fracture pattern divides the maxilla into two segments.
  - The lower segment, so-called the 'floating palate', contains:
    - The alveolus
    - The palate
    - The pterygoid plates.
- **Le Fort 2 fracture**
  - This is also known as a pyramidal fracture.
  - The fracture line passes:
    1 Across the nasal bones
    2 Into the medial wall of the orbit
    3 Diagonally downwards and outwards through the maxilla
    4 Through the pterygoid plates.
  - The bony fragment contains:
    - The lacrimal crests
    - The bulk of the maxilla
    - The piriform margin
    - The alveolus
    - The palate.
- **Le Fort 3 fracture**
  - This is also known as craniofacial dysjunction.
  - The fracture line passes:
    1 Through the nasofrontal (NF) suture
    2 Across the orbital floor to the ZF suture
    3 Through the zygomatic arch and pterygoid plates.
  - This results in detachment of the entire midfacial skeleton from the cranial base.
- Sagittal fractures of the maxilla and isolated fractures of the alveolus may also occur.
- Le Fort fracture patterns in the maxilla are often asymmetrical.

Symptoms and signs

Symptoms and signs of maxillary fractures include:

- Bruising and swelling
  - This is usually located superficially in the periorbital region and cheek.
  - Intra-oral bruising and swelling may also be present.
- Battle's sign
  - This is bruising over the mastoid process.
- Changes in dental occlusion
- Epistaxis
- Enophthalmos
- Diplopia
- Decreased sensation within the distribution of the inferior alveolar nerve
- A palpable step in the bone or dentition
  - The fracture segment is most commonly displaced downwards and posteriorly.
  - This results in a donkey- or dish-face appearance.
- Mobility of the maxillary segment
  - Mobility of the maxillary segment is the pathognomonic sign of a Le Fort fracture.
  - Clinically, it is demonstrated by stabilizing the glabella region with one hand while distracting the alveolus with the other.
  - Movement in the following areas helps differentiate the fracture pattern:
    1. Movement of the alveolus alone suggests a Le Fort 1 fracture.
    2. Movement of the alveolus and nasofrontal region suggests a Le Fort 2 fracture.
    3. Movement of the alveolus, nasofrontal region and ZF suture suggests a Le Fort 3 fracture.

Radiological investigation

The following radiological investigations can be used to identify the site, extent and displacement of zygomatic fractures.

- Plain films
  - PA views
  - Waters' views may demonstrate fracture lines or opacification of the maxillary sinus.
- Definitive investigation is by CT scan.
- A three-dimensional CT reconstruction may be useful in complex injuries.

Treatment

- OR&IF is the preferred method of treating Le Fort fractures.
- Access to the fracture lines can be gained through the following incisions.
  - A bicoronal incision, providing access to:
    - The nasofrontal region
    - The orbital walls
    - The ZF suture
    - The zygomatic arch.

- A lower-eyelid incision, providing access to:
  - The orbital floor
  - The infra-orbital rim.
- An upper buccal sulcus incision, providing access to:
  - The lower part of the maxilla.
- Open fixation is performed in the following way.

  1 Displaced fragments are reduced using Rowe's distraction forceps.

  2 The maxilla is stabilized by the application of IMF.

  3 Plates are then applied across the maxillary buttresses.

  4 Bone grafting may be required in:
  - Gaps resulting from missing bony segments.
  - Severely comminuted fractures.

3

Orbital fractures

- Orbital fractures often occur in conjunction with:
  - Zygomatic fractures
  - Nasoethmoid fractures
  - High Le Fort fractures.
- Isolated orbital fractures result from pressure applied to the globe.
- The orbit fractures at its weakest point, the inferomedial floor, known as the lamina papyracea (paper layer).

Symptoms and signs

Signs and symptoms of orbital fractures include:

- Bruising and swelling
- Subconjunctival haematoma with no posterior limit
- Palpable steps in the orbital margin
- Enophthalmos
  - Enophthalmos may be caused by:
    - Increase in the volume of the orbit as a result of the fracture.
    - Decrease in the volume of the orbital contents due to their herniation through the fracture line.
    - Tethering of orbital contents posteriorly in the fracture line.
    - Late enophthalmos may occur due to atrophy of intra-orbital fat.
- Diplopia
  - Diplopia may be caused by:
    - Entrapment of fat, fascial attachments or muscle within fracture lines.
    - Contusion of the recti or oblique muscles.
  - Diplopia usually occurs on upward gaze as most fractures and subsequent tethering occur inferiorly.

Radiological investigation

The following radiological investigations can be used to identify the site, extent and displacement of orbital fractures.

- Plain x-rays

- PA views
- Waters' views
- The 'tear drop' sign may be present, resulting from herniation of the orbital contents through the fracture line into the maxillary sinus.
- CT scan
  - Three-dimensional CT reconstruction may be indicated in complex injuries.

Indications for surgery

Surgery is usually performed in patients with:

- Symptomatic diplopia
- Significant enophthalmos
- Radiological evidence of orbital content entrapment
- Large bony defects
- Other fractures requiring fixation.

Surgical correction

- Orbital fractures are usually approached via lower-eyelid incisions.
- The orbital floor is explored to delineate the fractures.
- Any structures trapped within the fracture are released.
- The orbital floor is then reconstructed with one of the following:
  - Autologous tissue
    - Split calvarial bone graft
    - Rib
    - Iliac crest
    - A superficial segment of the anterior maxilla.
  - Alloplastic material
    - Titanium mesh
    - Gore-Tex
    - Silicone
    - Medpor wafers.

Nasal fractures

- The nose is the most commonly fractured facial bone.
- Lateral impacts result in deviation of the nasal bones and septum towards the opposite side.
- Frontal impacts result in:
  - Splaying of the nasal bones
  - Buckling or dislocation of the septum
  - Collapse of the nasal dorsum.

Classification

Stranc and Robertson have classified nasal fractures into the following groups:

- **Plane 1**
  - These injuries involve disruption of the cartilagenous septum.
  - The nasal bones are unaffected.

- **Plane 2**
  - These injuries involve disruption of the bony septum and the nasal bones.
- **Plane 3**
  - These injuries extend beyond the nasal skeleton into the piriform aperture and medial orbital rim.
  - They represent mild nasoethmoidal fractures.

Symptoms and signs

- Symptoms and signs of nasal fractures include:
  - Bruising and swelling
  - Obvious deformity.
- It is important to perform intranasal examination to exclude the presence of septal haematoma.
- If present, septal haematomas should be drained at their most dependent portion.
- Untreated haematomas may result in pressure necrosis of the nasal septum.

Treatment

- Simple fractures may be treated by closed reduction.
  1. Ashes' forceps are used to relocate the nasal septum.
  2. Walshams' forceps are used to relocate the nasal bones.
  3. The nose is then packed and an external splint applied.
- Secondary rhinoplasty may be required to correct late deformities.

Nasoethmoidal fractures

- Nasoethmoidal fractures are caused by trauma to the interorbital region.
- They often occur in conjunction with other facial fractures and involve:
  - The root of the nose
  - The medial wall of the orbit
  - The ethmoid air cells.

Symptoms and signs

Symptoms and signs of nasoethmoidal fractures include:

- Bruising and swelling
- A palpable bony step
- Telecanthus
  - This occurs if the medial canthal tendon is detached from its bony origin.
- Enophthalmos
- Diplopia.

Treatment

- Nasoethmoidal fractures are usually managed by OR&IF.
- Access to the fractures can be obtained via:
  - Overlying lacerations
  - Bicoronal incision
  - Medial orbital incisions (Lynch incision).

- The nasal bones are elevated and replaced in their anatomical position.
- A bone graft may be required to reconstruct the dorsum of the nose.
- The nasomaxillary buttress is reconstructed with plates and screws.
- The medial canthal tendon is exposed and reconstructed.
- The optimum method of medial canthal reconstruction depends on its bony attachment.
  - If the medial canthal tendon is attached to a large segment of bone, the bony fragment is secured into its anatomical position with a plate.
  - If the medial canthal tendon is attached to a small segment of bone, transnasal bony fixation is performed.
    - If the medial canthal tendon is avulsed or attached to a minute segment of bone, it is secured by transnasal wiring or with bone fixation devices.
- The lacrimal system is not routinely explored in patients with nasoethmoidal fractures, as most injuries are incomplete and settle within 6 weeks.

Frontal sinus fractures

The frontal sinus develops at approximately 6 years of age.

Symptoms and signs

Frontal sinus fractures may present with the following symptoms and signs:

- Bruising and swelling
- Palpable bony steps
- CSF rhinorrhoea.

Management

Indications for different forms of management are listed below.

- **Conservative management**
  - Undisplaced fracture of the anterior wall of the sinus
  - No CSF leak
  - Intact posterior wall
  - Unaffected drainage system.
- **OR&IF of the anterior wall of the sinus**
  - Displaced fracture of the anterior wall
  - No CSF leak
  - Intact posterior wall
  - Unaffected drainage system.
- **OR&IF of the anterior wall combined with obliteration of the frontal sinus**
  - Displaced fracture of the anterior wall
  - No CSF leak
  - Intact posterior wall
  - Damaged drainage system.
- **Cranialization of the frontal sinus**
  - Displaced fracture of the anterior wall
  - CSF leak

- Fracture of the posterior wall which is displaced less than the thickness of the bone
- Dural damage and hence the need of repair is rare in patients with minimal fracture displacement.

- **Cranialization of the frontal sinus with dural repair**
  - Displaced fracture of the anterior wall
  - CSF leak
  - Fracture of the posterior wall which is displaced more than the thickness of the bone

3

- Involvement of the drainage system is suspected if associated nasoethmoidal fractures are present.
- Obliteration of the frontal sinus is performed by:
  1 Complete removal of the mucosal lining the sinus
  2 Obliteration of the sinus by spontaneous osteogenesis or the insertion of a bone graft.
- Cranialization of the frontal sinus is achieved by:
  1 Complete removal of the mucosal lining the sinus
  2 Plugging of the nasofrontal duct with a bone graft
  3 Removing the posterior wall of the sinus
  4 Allowing the brain and dura to expand into the resultant dead space.

Complications

Potential complications of frontal sinus fractures are severe and include:

- Meningitis
- Cerebral abscesses
- Mucoceles
- Osteitis.

Oculoplastic surgery

Anatomy of the eyelid

- Each eyelid contains two lamellae:
  1 The external lamella is composed of skin and the orbicularis oculi muscle.
  2 The internal lamella is composed of the tarsal plate and conjunctiva.
- The levator palpebrae superioris muscle elevates the upper eyelid.
  - It originates in the apex of the orbit from the lesser wing of the sphenoid bone.
  - It passes forward and is tented over Whitnall's ligament.
  - Whitnall's ligament is a transverse structure which acts as a pulley converting the predominantly posterior pull of the muscle into vertical movement.
  - The levator palpebrae superioris terminates in the levator aponeurosis, which in turn inserts into:
    1 The tarsal plate posteriorly.
    2 The orbicularis oculi muscle and skin anteriorly.
  - In Caucasians, connections between the levator aponeurosis and the skin produce the upper eyelid fold.

- The upper eyelids of some Asian peoples differ from those of Caucasians in the following ways:
  1 The levator aponeurosis is solely attached to the tarsal plate, not to the skin or the orbicularis oculi muscle.
  2 The lids, therefore, do not have a fold.
  3 The orbital septum is attached lower on the anterior border of the tarsal plate.
  4 This allows the post-septal fat pads to herniate downwards anterior to the tarsal plate.
- Müller's muscle is a sympathetically innervated muscle originating from the underside of the levator muscle and inserting into the tarsal plate.
- The orbital septum originates from the bony periphery of the orbit and inserts onto the levator aponeurosis.
- Post-septal fat pads lie behind the orbital septum.
- There are two post-septal fat pads in the upper eyelid:
  1 The medial fat pad
  2 The central fat pad.
- There are three post-septal fat pads in the lower eyelid:
  1 The medial fat pad
  2 The central fat pad
  3 The lateral fat pad.
- Part, or all, of these fat pads is removed during traditional blepharoplasty.
- Preseptal fat pads lie between the orbital septum and the orbicularis oculi muscle.
  1 The retro-orbicularis oculi fat (ROOF) pad is in the upper eyelid.
  2 The suborbicularis oculi fat (SOOF) pad is in the lower eyelid.
- The lower eyelid has a similar structure to the upper eyelid.
- The retractor of the lower eyelid is known as the capsulopalpebral ligament and is continuous posteriorly with Lockwood's ligament.

Eyelid reconstruction

- Defects in the anterior and posterior lamella should be considered individually as each requires separate reconstruction.
- Excision of any lesion crossing the eyelid margin requires reconstruction of both lamellae.
- As a general rule, the lower eyelid is used to reconstruct the upper, but the upper is not used to reconstruct the lower.

Lower eyelid

Defects less than one-quarter of the horizontal width

- Lesions should be excised as a wedge or a pentagon and the defect closed in layers.
- Deep layers should be closed with absorbable 6/0 or 7/0 sutures.
- These should pass through the tarsal plate and just pick up the conjunctiva.

· They should then pass backwards through the conjunctiva and tarsal plate.
· The knot should be buried deeply within the eyelid anterior to the tarsal plate.
· The eyelid margin should be repaired with a non-absorbable 6/0 suture passing through the grey line.
· The grey line lies between the anterior and posterior lamellae on the eyelid margin.
· The eyelid skin should be closed with interrupted non-absorbable everting sutures.

Defects between one-quarter and one-third of the horizontal width

· The lesion should be excised as a wedge or a pentagon.
· A lateral cantholysis is then performed to mobilize the lower lid sufficiently to allow direct closure of the defect.
· Lateral cantholysis involves division of the lower limb of the lateral canthal tendon.
· It is performed in the following way:

1. Medial traction is applied to the lateral part of lower lid.
2. The lower limb of the lateral canthal tendon can then be felt as a tight band.
3. The lower limb is then dissected by spreading scissors along its edges.
4. It is then divided allowing the lower eyelid to advance medially.

Defects greater than one-third of the horizontal width

· These defects are usually repaired by a combination of:
  · A cheek-advancement flap to reconstruct the anterior lamella, and
  · A septomucosal graft to reconstruct the posterior lamella.
· Septomucosal grafts are harvested from the nasal septum.
· A lateral rhinotomy incision is usually required to gain adequate access to the septum.
· A lateral rhinotomy incision is a full-thickness incision in the alar groove.
· A strip of septum with overlying mucosa is harvested.
· Care is taken to preserve the integrity of the contralateral septal mucosa in order to avoid creating a septal perforation.
· The septomucosal graft is then scored and secured to the tarsal plates or canthal ligaments.
· A cheek-rotation flap is then advanced over the graft and secured.
· Superiorly, the mucosa of the septomucosal graft should slightly overlap the underlying graft so that the eyelid margin is reconstructed with mucosa.
· Cheek-advancement flaps may include a Z-plasty superiorly (McGregor pattern), alternatively it can be omitted (Mustardé pattern).

Alternatives for reconstructing the anterior lamella

· A Tripier flap from the upper lid can be transposed to the lower lid.
· Superiorly based transposition flaps from the cheek or lateral border of the nose are sometimes used to reconstruct the lower lid.
· Glabella flaps may be useful in reconstructing defects around the medial canthus.

Alternative for reconstructing the posterior lamella
The Hughes' tarsoconjunctival flap.

Upper eyelid

Defects less than one-third of the horizontal width
These defects are usually reconstructed by direct closure in a similar fashion to the lower eyelid.

Central full thickness defects greater than one-third of the horizontal width
- Central defects can be repaired with a Cutler–Beard flap.
- In this technique, the upper eyelid is reconstructed with an inferiorly based U-shaped flap taken from the lower eyelid.
- The apex of the flap lies approximately 5 mm below and parallel to the margin of the lower eyelid.
- The sides of the flap run vertically downwards from the apex.
- The flap is composed of the full thickness of the lower eyelid.
- The flap is advanced into the upper-eyelid defect under the 5 mm bridge of intact lower eyelid.
- It is sutured into position to lie across the globe.
- The eyelids are secured to each other by the flap for 6 weeks.
- The base of the flap lying across the globe is divided as a second procedure.

Alternative reconstructions
Mustardé lower-lid switch flaps combined with reconstruction of the lower lid are an alternative.
- In this technique, a laterally based transverse flap of the lower eyelid is transposed to the upper lid.
- It may be possible to directly close the lower-lid defect.
- If direct closure is not possible, the lower eyelid will need to be reconstructed separately by one of the techniques outlined above.
- The transposition flap from the lower eyelid is divided at a second procedure.

Ptosis
- Ptosis, or more correctly blepharoptosis, is drooping of the upper eyelid.
- It should be differentiated from the following.

Blepharophimosis
This condition is characterized by congenitally small palpebral fissures caused by the triad of:
1. Ptosis
2. Epicanthal folds
3. Telecanthus.

Blepharochalasis
This is excess eyelid skin seen in older individuals.

Blepharochalasis syndrome
- This condition usually occurs in young-to-middle-aged females and is of unknown aetiology.
- It is characterized by recurrent bouts of eyelid oedema.
- This results in excess eyelid skin and laxity of the canthi and lids.

Causes of eyelid ptosis
'MMAN'
- **M**yogenic:
  - Congenital levator dystrophy
  - Myasthenia gravis
  - Blepharophimosis.
- **M**echanical:
  - Blepharochalasis
  - Tumour
  - Scar.
- **A**poneurotic:
  - Congenital or acquired defects in the levator mechanism.
- **N**eurogenic:
  - Third nerve palsy
  - Horner's syndrome which consists of the following:
    1 Ptosis
    2 Meiosis
    3 Anhydrosis
    4 Enopthalmos.
  - Ptosis in Horner's syndrome is due to paralysis of the sympathetically innervated Müller's muscle.

Surgical correction
- The correct choice of operation is determined by:
  - The levator function
  - The degree of ptosis.
- The recommended operations are as follows:
  - Levator function >10 mm with ptosis <2 mm—Fasanella–Servat
  - Levator function >10 mm with ptosis <2 mm—aponeurosis surgery
  - Levator function <10 mm with ptosis <4 mm—levator resection
  - Levator function <10 mm with ptosis >4 mm—brow suspension.

Specific operations

Fasanella–Servat Müllerectomy
- The upper eyelid is everted.
- The conjunctiva and lower end of Müller's muscle are held in a clip.
- A longitudinal row of sutures is then placed through the conjunctiva and Müller's muscle just proximal to the clip.
- Conjunctiva and Müller's muscle distal to the line of sutures is excised.

Excision of a segment of the levator aponeurosis

- This can be performed via an anterior or posterior approach.
- The anterior approach passes through the skin of the upper eyelid.
- The posterior approach passes through the conjunctiva of the upper eyelid.
- Whichever approach is used, a transverse segment of levator aponeurosis is excised.
- The upper eyelid is raised by suturing the incised edges of the levator aponeurosis to one another.

Excision of a segment of the levator palpebrae superioris muscle

- This can be performed via an anterior or posterior incision.
- Beard has described an algorithm recommending width of levator resection.
- This varies from 10 to 23 mm depending on levator function and degree of ptosis.

Brow suspension

- In this procedure, a thin strip of fascia lata is inserted transversely across the upper lid just above its margin.
- The fascial strip is then tunnelled deep to the orbicularis oculi and frontalis muscles and secured to the periosteum of the forehead through small stab incisions.

Ectropion

Ectropion is movement of the lower-eyelid margin away from the globe.

Causes

'PICM'

- **P**aralytic
- **I**nvolutional
- **C**icatricial
- **M**echanical.

Surgical correction

- In cicatricial entropion, tethering structures should be released and the resultant defect reconstructed with a graft or a flap.
- Involutional ectropion is caused by laxity of the eyelid.
- The optimum method of correcting involutional ectropion depends on the site of maximum eyelid laxity and the stability of the canthal tendons.
  - If the site of maximum laxity is medial and the medial canthus is stable, a medial wedge excision should be performed.
  - If the site of maximum laxity is medial and the medial canthus is unstable, a medial canthopexy should be performed.
  - If the site of maximum laxity is lateral and the lateral canthus is stable, a Kuhnt–Szymanowski procedure should be performed.
  - If the site of maximum laxity is lateral and the lateral canthus is unstable, a lateral canthal sling procedure should be performed.

- Kuhnt–Szymanowski procedure
  - This technique combines:
    1 A blepharoplasty type lower-eyelid incision, and
    2 A wedge resection of the lateral part of the posterior lamella of the lower eyelid.
  - The blepharoplasty type incision provides better cosmesis than the alternative full-thickness lateral wedge excision.

- Lateral canthal sling
  - The lateral part of the lower lid can be tightened with a lateral canthal sling.
  - In this procedure, the lower limb of the lateral canthal tendon is dissected, tightened and secured to the lateral orbital rim.

Entropion

- Entropion is movement of the lower-eyelid margin towards the globe.
- Trauma to the globe from the lid margin and eyelashes results in pain and corneal scarring.

Causes

'CIC'

- **C**ongenital
- **I**nvolutional
- **C**icatricial.

Surgical correction

- Cicatricial entropion is caused by a vertical deficiency in the posterior lamella.
- It is treated by releasing the cicatricial bands and grafting the resultant defect.
- Numerous other operations to correct entropion have been described, including:
  - The use of everting sutures
  - Transverse fracture of the tarsal plate
  - Everting wedge excisions.

Other oculoplastic conditions

Trichiasis

- In this condition, the eyelashes are turned inwards towards the globe.
- It is often associated with entropion.

Symblepharon

- This is fusion of the eyelids to the globe.
- It is sometimes caused by chemical burns.

Epicanthic folds

- These are prominent vertical skin folds lying over the medial canthus.

- They occur in:
  - Patients with Down's syndrome
  - Patients with blepharophimosis
  - People of Asian descent.
- Prominent epicanthic folds may be released with a Mustardé jumping-man flap.
- The leg limbs of this flap should extend laterally onto the eyelids.

Evisceration
- This is removal of the contents of the globe, leaving the sclera intact.
- An acrylic implant is then placed inside the globe.
- A prosthesis is laid on top of the globe at a later date.

Enucleation
- This is removal of the globe, leaving the soft tissue of the orbit intact.
- The recti and oblique muscles may be sutured to the inserted implant so that they maintain their function.

Exenteration
- This is complete removal of:
  1. The contents of the orbit
  2. The eyelids.
- Exenteration is performed by dissection in a subperiosteal plane.
- The resultant defect can be left to heal by secondary intention which can take up to 3 months.
- Alternatively, the exenteration defect can be reconstructed with the following local flaps:
  - Cervicofacial flaps
  - Forehead flaps
  - Scalp flaps
  - Flaps from the temporal region.

Facial palsy

Anatomy of the facial nerve
- The facial nerve supplies structures derived from the second branchial arch.
- It is the 7th cranial nerve and is motor to the muscles of facial expression.
- It originates in the pontine region of the brain stem and enters the temporal bone at the internal auditory meatus alongside the 8th cranial nerve.
- In its intratemporal course, the facial nerve gives off the following branches:
  1. Greater petrosal nerve
     - This is the nerve of tear secretion.
     - It is secretomotor to the lacrimal gland and the glands of the palate.
  2. Tympanic nerve
     - This is a small sensory branch.

3 Nerve to stapedius

- The stapedius muscle acts to dampen loud noises.

4 Chorda tympani

- This nerve supplies taste to the anterior two-thirds of the tongue.
- It travels with the lingual nerve to reach the tongue.

- The facial nerve exits the temporal bone at the stylomastoid foramen.
- Clinically, it may be possible to differentiate sites of facial nerve injuries.
- Patients with injuries at, or distal to, the stylomastoid foramen have paralysis of the facial musculature.
- Patients with more proximal injuries in the brain or in the temporal bone have the following additional symptoms:
  - Loss of taste in the anterior two-thirds of the tongue (due to damage to the chorda tympani).
  - Hyperacusia (due to damage to the nerve to stapedius).
- The first branch of the facial nerve after it exits the stylomastoid foramen is the posterior auricular nerve, which supplies the occipital muscles and sensation to a small area behind the ear lobe.
- The next branch is a muscular branch supplying the posterior belly of the digastric and stylohyoid muscles.
- Distal to these branches, the facial nerve divides into:

1 An upper temporozygomatic branch

2 A lower cervicofacial branch.

Within the substance of the parotid gland, each branch divides and rejoins only to divide again into the following five terminal branches:

1 Temporal or frontal branch

- This travels along Pitanguy's line.
- This line extends from 0.5 cm below the tragus to 1.5 cm above and lateral to the eyebrow.
- The frontal branch becomes increasingly superficial as it travels upwards.
- It lies just deep to the temporoparietal (superficial temporal) fascia in the temple.
- Lower motor-neurone lesions of the facial nerve, or its frontal branch, result in paralysis of the ipsilateral frontalis muscle.

2 Zygomatic branch

- This nerve divides into branches supplying the orbicularis oculi muscle.
- Division results in inability to close the eye.

3 Buccal branch

- This nerve divides into multiple branches which travel alongside the parotid duct.
- These branches supply the buccinator muscle and the muscles of the upper lip.
- Division of these branches causes difficulty in emptying the cheek.

4 Marginal mandibular branch

- This nerve runs just below the border of the mandible deep to the platysma muscle and superficial to the facial vein.
- The mandibular branch supplies the muscles of the lower lip.
- Division of this nerve result in elevation of the corner of the mouth.

5 Cervical branch

- This nerve runs downwards into the neck to supply the platysma muscle.

- **Buccal and zygomatic branches**
  - There is a significant degree of crossover between the buccal and zygomatic branches of the facial nerve.
  - Injury to either of these nerves is often compensated for by growth from the other.
  - There is little crossover from adjacent nerves to the frontal and marginal mandibular branches.
  - Injuries to these nerves are seldom compensated by cross-innervation from adjacent branches.

Congenital causes

Congenital causes of facial nerve paralysis include the following.

Möbius syndrome

- This syndrome typically involves paralysis of the 6th and 7th cranial nerves and is characterized by bilateral facial paralysis.
- The 3rd, 5th, 9th and 12th cranial nerves may also be involved.
- Limb abnormalities are present in 25% of cases.
- Pectoral abnormalities are present in 15% of cases.

Goldenhar's syndrome

- Patients with this syndrome have:
  1. Hemifacial microsomia
  2. The presence of epibulbar dermoids.
- In some cases the facial nerve may also be abnormal.

Acquired causes

Acquired causes of facial nerve palsy can be subdivided by the sites at which they occur.

- Central causes include:
  - Tumours
  - Multiple sclerosis
  - Polio.
- Intratemporal causes include:
  - Bell's palsy
  - Trauma
  - Otitis media
  - Cholesteatoma
  - Acoustic neuroma
  - Herpes zoster oticus (Ramsay Hunt syndrome).
- Extratemporal causes include:
  - Trauma
  - Parotid malignancy
  - Iatrogenic injury.

Bell's palsy

- This syndrome was first described by Charles Bell in 1814.
- Originally, it referred to facial nerve paralysis from any cause.
- Today, the term is used to describe idiopathic facial nerve paralysis.
- Bell's palsy is diagnosed by exclusion once other acquired causes of facial nerve paralysis have been eliminated.
- Bell's palsy may be caused by a viral infection producing swelling of the facial nerve within its tight intratemporal course.
- Most patients with Bell's palsy recover full facial nerve function.
- Those who go on to recover completely usually show some return of facial movement within 4 weeks.
- In severe cases, complete axonal degeneration occurs.
- In these patients, recovery usually begins after 3 months and may be incomplete.

Grading

House and Brackman have described the following grading system for facial palsy.

- *Grade 1*: some mimetic (spontaneous) movement.
- *Grade 2*: no mimetic movement.
- *Grade 3*: only mass action of the facial muscles.
- *Grade 4*: the patient is unable to completely close their eyelids.
- *Grade 5*: the face remains symmetrical despite complete facial paralysis.
- *Grade 6*: an asymmetrical face with no movement.

Symptoms and signs

- When examining patients with facial paralysis, it is important to look for:
  - Asymmetry
  - Scars or signs of previous trauma
  - Absence of forehead wrinkles
  - Position and movement of the upper eyelid
  - Condition of the conjunctiva for evidence of exposure
  - Ectropion of the lower eyelid
  - Position of the mouth.
- It is important to:
  - Test the strength of eyelid closure
  - Perform the lower-eyelid snap test (see p. 293)
  - Assess whether the patient has any nasal valving
  - Verify that the temporalis muscle is contracting by palpating it as the patient clenches their jaw.

Special tests

The following tests help in locating the site of the facial nerve lesion.

- Schirmer's test
  - This test assesses the integrity of the greater petrosal nerve by measuring tear secretion.

- A strip of specially designed filter paper is placed in the lower conjunctiva for 5 min.
- <10 mm of wetting during this time is considered abnormal.
- Local anaesthetic can be added to the eye to block reflex tear secretion.
- If local anaesthetic is added, the test is known as Schirmer's test 2.
- The stapedius reflex test
  - This test assesses the integrity of the facial nerve branch to the stapedius muscle.
- Taste to the anterior two-thirds of tongue
  - This test assesses the integrity of the chorda tympani.

Treatment

- Treatment of facial nerve palsy may be: (i) non-operative; or (ii) operative.
- Operative techniques may be: (i) static; or (ii) dynamic.

Non-operative treatment

- Protection of the eye is of paramount importance.
- The eye can be protected by:
  - Regular use of lubricating eye drops
  - Wearing glasses
  - Taping the eyelids closed at night.
- Paralytic ectropion may be helped by:
  - Horizontal taping of the lower eyelids.
- Botulinum toxin
  - Recently, there have been reports of the use of the toxin produced by the bacteria *Clostridium botulinum* (Botox) in the treatment of facial palsy.
  - When injected Botox produces paralysis of the facial musculature by interfering with the release of acetylcholine from motor nerve endplates.
  - Botox injections into the normal side of the face may improve facial symmetry.

Operative treatment

Static procedures

- Static procedures around the eye include:
  - **Temporary tarsorrhaphy**
    - Tarsorrhaphies narrow the palpebral fissure by joining a portion of the eyelids to one another.
    - Narrowing the palpebral fissure aids eye closure.
    - Temporary tarsorrhaphy is usually performed when there is some expectation of recovery.
  - **Permanent tarsorrhaphy**
    - Permanent tarsorrhaphy is usually performed when there is little expectation of recovery.
  - **Kuhnt–Szymanowski split-level eyelid resection**
    - This operation is used to correct paralytic ectropion of the lower eyelid (see p. 144).

- **Insertion of gold weights or springs**
  - These can be inserted into the upper eyelid to help eye closure.
- **Brow lifts**
  - Brow lifts can be performed via an endoscopic or open approach.
  - They elevate the ptotic brow caused by paralysis of the frontalis muscle.
- **Forehead skin excision**
  - Depending on the site of maximum ptosis, skin excisions may be performed above the eyebrow or in the temple.

- Static procedures around the mouth include:
  - **Unilateral face lift type procedures**
    - These operations are used to remove skin excess and improve facial symmetry.
  - **Static slings**
    - Segments of fascia lata can be used to elevate the corner of the mouth and nose.

Dynamic procedures

Dynamic procedures to improve the appearance of patients with facial palsy include:

- **Nerve repair**
  - Direct repair can be performed on damaged or cut nerves.
  - In optimal conditions, direct nerve repair is associated with good recovery of function.
- **Primary nerve grafting**
  - This technique is used after nerve resection during tumour removal.
  - Branches of the cervical plexus or the sural nerve are used as grafts to bridge the defect.
- **Cross-facial nerve grafting**
  - This technique was described by Scaramella in 1970.
  - A sural nerve graft is anastamosed to:
    - A branch of the facial nerve on the unaffected side of the face
    - The distal stump of the facial nerve branches on the affected side of the face
  - Cross-facial nerve grafting can be performed as a one- or two-stage procedure.
  - In the two-stage procedure, a nerve graft is inserted across the face in the first operation.
  - Growth of axons is assessed by an advancing Tinel's sign.
  - The second operation is performed when nerve regeneration has advanced sufficiently.
  - In the second operation, the terminal neuroma is resected and the end of the graft is sutured to the distal stump of the facial nerve.
  - Despite initial enthusiasm, cross-facial nerve grafting has enjoyed only limited success.
  - This is because the ability of the facial musculature to re-innervate decreases with time.

- **Nerve transfers**
  - The following nerves can be transferred onto the distal stump of the facial nerve.
    - The glossopharyngeal nerve
    - The hypoglossal nerve
    - The accessory nerve
    - The phrenic nerve
  - Nerve transfers have the following advantages.
    - They are relatively easy to perform.
    - Unlike a nerve graft, they require nerve regeneration over a single suture line.
  - However, they have the following disadvantages.
    - They tend to produce coarse, uncoordinated facial movements.
    - Function of donor nerve is lost.
  - Hypoglossal nerve transfer is sometimes used after excision of a segment of facial nerve during tumour resection.
- **Local muscle flaps**

The following local and regional muscles can be transferred to mimic facial movement:

  - The masseter muscle
    - Part, or all, of the masseter muscle can be transferred.
    - In this procedure the muscle is divided into three slips and inserted: (i) above the lip; (ii) into the commissure, and; (iii) below the lip
  - The temporalis muscle
    - The temporalis muscle can be transposed and inserted around the eye and mouth.
    - Additional periosteal extensions or fascial grafts are usually necessary to elongate the muscle.
  - The sternocleidomastoid muscle
    - This transfer has been described but is seldom indicated.
- **Cross-facial nerve grafting combined with free-muscle transfer**

In suitable patients, the combination of these procedures offers the best hope of restoring voluntary movement to the face but, due to poor axonal regeneration, the success of this technique decreases with age. One- and two-stage procedures have been described.

  - *One-stage procedure*
    - The muscle is harvested with its motor nerve, is transferred to the face, and its motor nerve is sutured to a branch of the facial nerve.
  - Advantages of the one-stage operation:
    - The axons only have to regenerate over a single suture line.
    - A nerve graft is not required and no donor defect results.
    - A second operation is avoided.
  - Disadvantages of the one-stage operation:
    - The relative lack of suitable muscles with a nerve of sufficient length does not permit one-stage transfer.
    - The transferred muscle remains denervated for a longer period than in the two-stage procedure.

- *Two-stage procedure*

  1 A sural nerve graft is harvested, the graft is then reversed and tunnelled across the upper lip just below the anterior nasal spine. The graft is anastomosed to a branch of the facial nerve on the functioning side of the face, with the free end secured anterior to the tragus on the affected side. The nerve graft is reversed in an effort to minimize axonal growth up its side branches and away from the main trunk. Axonal growth across the face is monitored by an advancing Tinel's sign.

  2 Once nerve regeneration has progressed sufficiently, the second operation is performed. A free-muscle flap is harvested, and the muscle is inserted proximally onto the zygomatic arch and distally around the mouth and nose. Positioning aims to replicate the line of pull of the zygomaticus major muscle. The neuroma at the end of the nerve graft is resected and the distal end of the graft is sutured to the motor nerve of the muscle.
- The following muscles are commonly used as free transfers for facial reanimation.
  - The gracilis muscle
  - The pectoralis minor muscle
  - The latissimus dorsi muscle.
- Each has its advocates but none completely simulates the subtle mimetic movements of the face.

Treatment of Möbius syndrome

- As the contralateral facial nerve is abnormal, it cannot be used as a donor to innervate the face.
- Other donor motor nerves must therefore be used to innervate any free muscle transfer.
- This can be achieved by:
  - Transposing a nerve
  - Use of an interposition nerve graft.
- The following nerves have been used to power free-tissue transfers:
  - A portion of the ipsilateral accesary nerve
  - The trigeminal nerve
  - The ipsilateral hypoglossal nerve is often abnormal and therefore not suitable as a donor motor nerve.

Abnormalities of the ear

Embryology

- The external ear begins to form at the 4th week of gestation.
- By 6 weeks it is comprised of:
  - Three anterior hillocks derived from the first branchial arch.
  - Three posterior hillocks derived from the second branchial arch.
- Between the two lie:
  - The first branchial cleft externally.
  - The first pharyngeal pouch internally.

- The first branchial cleft develops into the external auditory meatus.
- The hillocks differentiate into the following structures.
  1 Lower anterior hillock—the tragus
  2 Middle anterior hillock—the crus of the helix
  3 Upper anterior hillock—the major portion of the helix
  4 Lower posterior hillock—the lobule and the lower part of the helix
  5 Middle posterior hillock—the antitragus
  6 Upper posterior hillock—the antihelix.

The surface anatomy of the ear

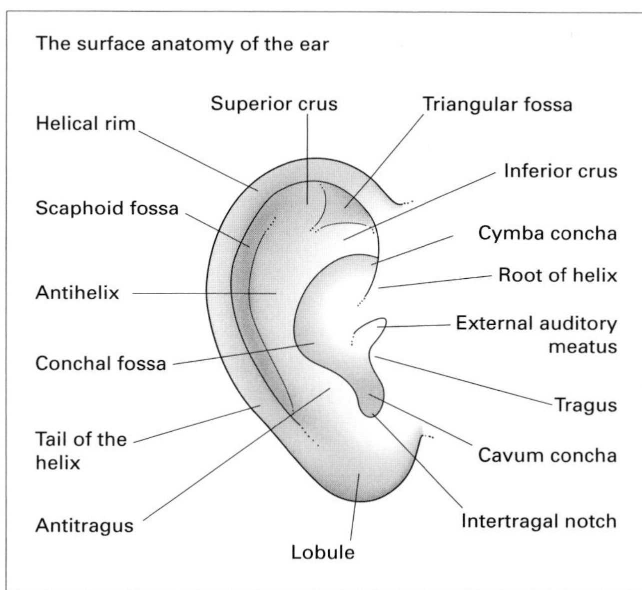

Blood supply

The ear is supplied by the following arteries.

- The posterior auricular artery
  - This is a branch of the external carotid artery.
  - It runs upwards in the sulcus behind the ear.
  - It supplies blood to the posterior skin of the ear and the lobule.
- The superficial temporal artery
  - This is a terminal branch of the external carotid artery.
  - It runs upwards just in front of the ear alongside the auriculotemporal nerve.
  - It supplies blood to the lateral aspect of the ear.
- The occipital artery
  - This is the dominant supply to the posterior ear in approximately 10% of people.

Nerve supply

The following nerves supply sensation to the ear.

- Greater auricular nerve
  - This nerve supplies sensation to the inner and outer aspects of the lower half of the ear.
- Auriculotemporal nerve
  - This nerve supplies sensation to the outer aspect of the superior half of the ear.
- Lesser occipital nerve
  - This nerve supplies sensation to the inner aspect of the superior half of the ear.
- Auricular branch of the vagus nerve
  - This is also known as the Alderman's nerve.
  - It supplies sensation to the conchal fossa and the external auditory meatus.
  - Stimulation of this nerve, by applying cold and then warm water to the conchal fossa, induces vagal-induced vomiting.

Classification

Tanzer has classified auricular deformities into the following groups.

- *Type 1*: anotia
- *Type 2*: microtia with atresia of the external auditory meatus
- *Type 2B*: microtia without atresia of the external auditory meatus
- *Type 3*: hypoplasia of the middle-third of the ear
- *Type 4*: constricted ear
- *Type 4B*: cryptotia
- *Type 4C*: hypoplasia of the entire upper-third of the ear
- *Type 5*: prominent ear

Anotia

- Anotia is complete absence of the ear.
- The incidence of anotia is:
  - One in 6000 in the Western world
  - One in 4000 in Japan
  - One in 1000 in Navajo Indians.

Syndromes associated with anotia

- Treacher Collins syndrome
  - Anotia is usually bilateral.
- Hemifacial microsomia
  - Anotia is usually unilateral.

Reconstruction

- The ear has attained approximately 85% of its adult size by the time a child is 4 years of age.

- The rib cartilages are large enough to permit fabrication of an adult-sized ear by the time the child is 6 years of age.

Ear reconstruction is performed in the following way.

- **Stage one**
  1. The contours of the normal ear are traced onto an x-ray sheet.
  2. Assessing the correct position for the new ear
     - The x-ray pattern is placed in a similar position to the contralateral ear.
  3. Fabrication of the cartilaginous framework of the ear
     - The helical rim can be fashioned from the costal cartilage of the first contralateral floating rib (usually the 8th).
     - The base of the ear can be fashioned from the synchondrosis between the contralateral 6th and 7th costal cartilages.
     - A wood carving chisel is used to sculpture the cartilaginous framework, designed with an exaggerated helical rim.
     - Allogenic cartilage, silicone or medpor have also been used to fabricate a framework (allogenic cartilage is prone to reabsorbtion and alloplastic polymers to extrusion).
  4. Creation of a subcutaneous pocket
     - A subcutaneous pocket is created at the site of the new ear.
     - The pocket is dissected through an incision anterior to the auricular vestige.
     - Any residual cartilage is removed.
     - The cartilaginous framework is then inserted into the pocket.
     - Suction drains are positioned in the pocket to prevent fluid accumulation.
     - In post-traumatic cases or when there has been extensive previous surgery dissection of the pocket may be difficult.
     - In these patients, a temporoparietal fascial flap can be used to cover the auricular framework.
- **Stage two**
  - The lobule is rotated from its anterior position into its correct anatomical site.
- **Stage three**
  - A sulcus is created behind the reconstructed ear.
    - An incision is made just outside the helical rim.
    - 2–4 mm of posterior auricular skin is then advanced onto the helical rim.
    - The sulcus is reconstructed with a thick split-thickness skin graft.

Otoplasty

Otoplasty is a term for prominent ear correction.

- Prominent ears can be corrected by:
  - Suture techniques
  - Excisional techniques
  - Cartilage moulding techniques.
- A combination of techniques can be used.
- There have been reports from Japan of the successful treatment of prominent ears with splints applied early in life.

Suture techniques

Concha–mastoid sutures

· These sutures pass between the cartilage of the posterior aspect of the conchal fossa and the fascia overlying the mastoid process.
· They pull the conchal fossa towards the head reducing the prominence of the ear.

Mustardé sutures

· These mattress sutures pass through the cartilage of the scaphoid and conchal fossas.
· They increase the degree of antihelical folding.

Fossa-fascia sutures

· These mattress sutures pass between the scaphoid fossa and the temporal fascia.
· They are primarily used to correct prominence of the upper part of the ear.

Excisional techniques

Skin excision alone

· Excision of posterior skin without correction of the cartilagenous defect almost inevitably results in recurrence of the deformity.
· The following patterns of skin excision can be used to correct a prominent lobule.
  · Incorporating a fish-tail pattern at the lower end of the posterior skin incision.
  · Making a transverse incision, which is then closed vertically, on the posterior aspect of the lobule.

Excision of a portion of conchal fossa

· Conchal fossa excisions alone can be used in patients with:
  · Deep conchal fossas
  · Normal antihelical folds.
· Conchal fossa excision may be performed through an anterior or posterior incision.

Cartilage moulding techniques

· Cartilage moulding can be performed by:
  · Open scoring after exposure of the cartilage.
  · Closed techniques in which the cartilage is scored through a small anterior or posterior skin incision.
· Both techniques rely on the Gibson principle which states that cartilage bends away from a scored surface.
· The moulded cartilage can be secured in its new position with sutures.

Specific congenital abnormalities

The constricted ear

- This is characterized by deficiency in the circumference of the helix.
- The deformity is difficult to correct.
- It is usually managed with the combination of a cartilage moulding and a suture technique of otoplasty.

Stahl's ear

- This deformity is characterized by the presence of an abnormal third crus which radially transverses the superior third of the ear.
- Correction is difficult and may require a combination of excision, scoring and a suture technique of otoplasty.

Cryptotia

- In this rare congenital deformity part of the ear is buried beneath the skin of the scalp.
- It is common in Japan where it has an incidence of one in 400.
- Surgery involves elevating the ear and creating a posterior sulcus with skin grafts or flaps.

Reconstructing the amputated ear

Many methods of treating traumatic amputation of the ear have been described, including:

- Replacement of the amputated segment as a composite graft
  - Composite grafts are unlikely to take if >1.5 cm in diameter.
- Techniques aimed at increasing take of an amputated segment replaced as a composite graft include:
  - Removal of the superficial layer of the ear by excision or dermabrasion
    - The denuded segment is then reattached to the ear remnant and buried in a subcutaneous pocket behind the ear.
  - Removal of the posterior skin of the ear and fenestration of the cartilage
    - A section of posterior auricular skin is excised and the composite graft is inset into this area.
    - The sulcus is reconstructed at a second operation.
  - Dermabrasion of the amputated segment and immediate coverage with a temporoparietal fascia flap covered with a skin graft.
- Microsurgical ear replantation
  - When possible, this is the optimum method of reconstructing an amputated ear.
  - If no suitable veins are found, artery-only replantation can be performed.
  - Subsequent venous congestion of the amputated segment can be relieved by the application of leeches.
- Banking of the cartilagenous framework of the amputated segment of the ear

- This technique preserves the cartilagenous framework for later use during delayed reconstruction.
- Deformity and atrophy of the banked cartilage limit the use of this technique.

Vascular abnormalities

Classification

- Mulliken and Glowacki have classified vascular abnormalities into: (i) haemangiomas; and (ii) vascular malformations.
- Haemangiomas are not usually present at birth but rapidly increase in size before involuting.
- Vascular malformations are present at birth and grow in proportion to body size.
- The classification is useful in that it aids:
  - Diagnosis
  - Planning
  - Management
  - Predicting the future behaviour of lesions.

Haemangiomas

Incidence

- Haemangiomas are the most common tumour of infancy.
- They occur more frequently in premature babies.
- Females are three times as likely to be affected as males.
- Haemangiomas are not usually present at birth.
- 80% are noticed within the 1st month of life.
- 60% occur in the head and neck.

Clinical behaviour

- The cycle of growth and involution of haemangiomas has been classified into the following seven stages.
  - *Stage 1*: origin (Herald patch)
  - *Stage 2*: initial growth
  - *Stage 3*: intermediate growth
  - *Stage 4*: completed growth
  - *Stage 5*: initial involution
  - *Stage 6*: intermediate involution
  - *Stage 7*: completed involution.
- The haemangioma is in its proliferative phase during stages 1–4.
- This phase typically lasts between 6 and 18 months.
- The haemangioma is in its involutional phase during stages 5–7.
- This phase typically starts between 6 and 18 months of age.
- It is usually complete by the time the child is 9 years of age.

· The following is a rough guide to the age at which a haemangioma can be expected to have resolved.
  · 60% by 6 years of age
  · 70% by 7 years of age
  · 80% by 8 years of age
  · 90% by 9 years of age.
· Haemangiomas do not usually completely disappear.
· Some fibro-fatty swelling usually remains at the site of the haemangioma.
· Haemangiomas in areas such as the lip and oral mucosa tend to undergo less regression than those at other sites.

Clinical characteristics

· In the proliferative phase, haemangiomas are bright red with slightly bosselated surfaces.
· Due to this appearance, haemangiomas are also known as 'strawberry naevi'.
· Their consistency is soft and doughy.
· If haemangiomas are located deeply in the subcutaneous tissue, they can take on a bluish tinge.
· Deeply located lesions are sometimes called cavernous haemangiomas.
· As the haemangioma involutes, it develops grey patches.
· These patches gradually enlarge as the colour of the haemangioma gradually fades.

Histological appearance

· Histologically, haemangiomas are characterized by plump hyperplastic vascular endothelium.
· This endothelium contains up to 40 times the normal number of mast cells.
· Some authorities believe that heparin secreted by these cells plays central a role in the pathogenesis of haemangiomas.
· Endothelial turnover is extremely rapid and can take as little as 24 h.

Complications

These can be subdivided into those: (i) intrinsic to the haemangioma; and (ii) due to obstruction of a body orifice.

Intrinsic complications

Bleeding

· Bleeding from a haemangioma is rare and is usually caused by trauma.

Ulceration

· Ulceration usually occurs in areas such as the perineum in which the haemangioma is subject to repeated trauma.
· Ulceration can lead to scarring.

Infection

· Infection usually occurs secondary to ulceration.

Kasabach–Merritt phenomenon

· This is a rare, life-threatening condition caused by platelet trapping within the haemangioma.

· This results in a consumptive coagulopathy.

· The peak incidence of this condition is at about 5 weeks of age.

· It usually presents as swelling and bruising adjacent to the haemangioma.

· It should be managed in a paediatric intensive care setting.

Obstructive complications

Visual obstruction

· Obstruction of the visual axis of the eye can result in amblyopia and anisometropia in as little as one week.

· Amblyopia is permanent visual loss due to a central malfunction in the visual cortex.

· It is not correctable by refraction.

· Anisometropia is the permanent loss of binocular vision due to a central malfunction in the visual cortex.

· Direct pressure on the globe from a haemangioma can produce strabismus.

· Obstruction of the visual axis requires urgent treatment.

· This normally consists of the administration of high-dose oral steroids.

· If no improvement is seen within a week, surgical debulking is sometimes necessary.

Airway obstruction

· Haemangiomas may obstruct the airway.

· Glottic lesions may present with biphasic stridor.

· Enlarging lesions are usually managed with surgical resection.

External acoustic meatus obstruction

· This is uncommon and can result in conductive deafness.

Treatment

· Haemangiomas are usually treated conservatively as the vast majority involute satisfactorily without intervention.

· Indications for treatment include:
  · Significant obstruction of the visual axis, airway or auditory canal
  · Ulceration or haemorrhage due to local trauma
  · The Kasabach–Merritt phenomenon
  · Aesthetic considerations.

· Treatment may be non-invasive or invasive.

3

Non-invasive treatments

Systemic steroids

- Systemic steroids are usually used in short courses at doses of 2 mg/kg/day.
- Treatment results in some degree of involution in 50–90% of cases.
- Very high doses of steroids are occasionally used to treat patients with the Kasabach–Merritt phenomenon.

Interferon alpha 2a

- This is administered subcutaneously.
- Interferon (IF) alpha 2a is not usually given at the same time as steroids.
- Treatment with IF alpha 2a is usually reserved for life-threatening conditions such as hepatic haemangiomas and the Kasabach–Merritt phenomenon.

Antiplatelet drugs

Aspirin has been used for its antiplatelet action in patients with the Kasabach–Merritt phenomenon.

Compression, radiotherapy and chemotherapy

- These have been advocated in the past but have not gained universal acceptance.

Invasive treatments

Intralesional steroid injection

- This method of administering steroids is associated with a high rate of local complications.
- Local injection does not avoid systemic absorption.
- Steroids are usually administered systemically rather than locally.

Intralesional OK-432 injection

- This new compound is derived from denatured streptococcal protein.
- It is believed to act as an immunological stimulant causing regression of the haemangioma.

Intralesional injection of sclerosing agents

- Intralesional injections of hypertonic saline sotradecol and glucose have been used to treat haemangiomas.

Surgical debulking

- Surgical debulking of haemangiomas is sometimes indicated particularly for lesions around the eye.
- Nasal haemangiomas are often best approached via an open rhinoplasty approach.

Laser treatment

- Laser treatment can be performed:
  - Externally on the surface of the haemangioma
  - Internally via a fibreoptic cable inserted into the lesion.
- There is some evidence that pulse dye laser treatment may prevent progression of haemangiomas if given early enough.

Selective embolization

Selective embolization of haemangiomas has met with limited success.

Vascular malformations

- Unlike haemangiomas, vascular malformations are not tumours.
- They occur as a result of faulty embryological development.
- Vascular malformations are present at birth and grow in proportion to the body.

Classification

Vascular malformations are classified into: (i) low-flow lesions; and (ii) high-flow lesions.

Low-flow lesions

Capillary malformations

- Capillary malformations are also known as port-wine stains.
- They commonly occur within the distribution of the trigeminal nerve.
- They are usually flat and pale in youth, becoming increasingly raised, nodular and darker as the patient ages.
- Capillary malformations are usually treated with the pulse dye laser.
- Waner has described the following grading system for capillary malformations:
  - *Grade 1*: sparse, pale, non-confluent discoloration
  - *Grade 2*: denser pink non-confluent discoloration
  - *Grade 3*: discrete ectatic vessels
  - *Grade 4*: a confluent patch
  - *Grade 5*: a nodular lesion.

Venous malformations

- Venous malformations are present at birth although they may not be noticed until the child is older.
- They usually present as:
  - A faint-blue patch
  - A soft-blue compressible mass.
- Venous malformations are often incorrectly labelled as cavernous haemangiomas.
- Venous malformations are usually solitary and tend to occur in cutaneous or visceral locations.
- They may be very large.
- They are easily compressible and swell when dependent.

- They may contain phleboliths and thrombosis can occur within them.
- Treatment is indicated on functional or aesthetic grounds and may consist of:
  - Intralesional sclerotherapy with 100% ethanol or Ethibloc (a mixture of zein, a corn protein, alcohol and contrast medium)
  - Surgical resection
  - A combination of surgical resection and sclerotherapy.

Lymphatic malformations

- Lymphatic malformations may be:
  - Microcystic
  - Macrocystic
  - Mixed micro- and macrocystic
- Lymphangiomas are microcystic lymphatic malformations.
- Cystic hygromas are macrocystic lymphatic malformations.
- Lymphangioma circumscriptum is characterized by the presence of small intradermal vesicles overlying a deeper lymphatic malformation.
- Most lymphatic malformations are present at birth or appear within the first 2 years of life.
- Lymphatic malformations do not usually involute spontaneously.
- They tend to expand and contract depending on the movement of lymphatic fluid.
- Lymphatic malformations may enlarge if:
  - They become infected
  - Bleeding occurs within them.
- Sudden enlargement should be managed conservatively with analgesia and antibiotics.
- Lymphatic malformations can be treated with intralesional injection of OK-432.
- Lymphatic malformations tend to recur if not fully excised.
- Surgery is often complicated by delayed wound healing.

High-flow lesions

Arterial malformations

- Pure arterial malformations include:
  - Aneurysms
  - Stenosis
  - Tortuous arteries
  - Arteries following an abnormal course.
- Arterial malformations rarely occur as isolated abnormalities.

Arteriovenous malformations

- Arteriovenous malformations (AVMs) are usually present at birth but only become clinically apparent in infancy or childhood.
- Trauma or puberty triggers expansion, manifested by:
  - Darkening of the lesion

- Enlargement of the lesion
- Development of a bruit and thrill.
- Sequelae of expansion include:
  - Ischaemic skin changes
  - Ulceration
  - Bleeding
  - Pain
  - Increased cardiac output.

- The following staging system of AVMs has been described by Schobinger:
  - *Stage 1*: a blue skin-blush.
  - *Stage 2*: a mass associated with a bruit and a thrill.
  - *Stage 3*: a mass associated with ulceration, bleeding and pain.
  - *Stage 4*: stage 3 lesions producing heart failure.

Treatment

- AVMs are notoriously difficult to treat.
- Principles of management include:

1 Accurate diagnosis by angiography to localize the supplying vessels.
2 Preoperative correction of any clotting abnormalities.
3 Preoperative embolization.
4 Attempts to resect the whole lesion.
5 Minimization of intra-operative bleeding by use of hypotensive anaesthesia, quilting mattress sutures and circulatory arrest and diversion if necessary.
6 Reconstruction of the defect.

- AVMs are usually treated when endangering signs arise (stages 3 and 4).
- The value of earlier treatment during stages 2 and 3 is contentious.
- Ligation, or embolization, of proximal feeding vessels is absolutely contraindicated as it increases collateral supply, resulting in enlargement of the lesion
- Embolization followed by resection within 24–72 h is the treatment of choice for symptomatic AVMs.
- Embolization should be performed into the nidus of the malformation.
- AVMs should be completely excised back to normal tissue.
- Limits of resection can be gauged by:
  - Preoperative MRI scanning
  - Angiography
  - Intra-operative Doppler studies
  - Frozen sections
  - The pattern of bleeding at the wound edge.

Syndromes associated with vascular lesions

The following syndromes are associated with vascular lesions.

Sturge–Weber syndrome

- This syndrome is characterized by port-wine stains within the distribution of the opthalmic and maxillary branches of the trigeminal nerve.

- It is associated with:
  - Meningeal vascular malformations
  - Motor seizures, including epilepsy
  - A low IQ
  - Eye abnormalities, including glaucoma.

Klippel–Trenaunay syndrome

- This syndrome is characterized by a port-wine stain of an extremity (usually the leg).
- Beneath the port-wine stain lies a venous or lymphatic malformation.
- An abnormal lateral vein may be present.
- The lateral vein should not be removed or ligated as it may be the only vessel providing venous drainage from the limb.
- Limb hypertrophy with bony enlargement may occur.

Parkes–Weber syndrome

- This syndrome is similar to Klippel–Trenaunay syndrome except that affected patients also have an arteriovenous fistula.

Osler–Weber–Rendu syndrome

- This syndrome is also known as hereditary haemorrhagic telangiectasia.
- It is inherited in an autosomal dominant fashion and is characterized by the presence of bright red AVMs in the:
  - Skin
  - Mucous membranes
  - Lungs
  - Abdominal viscera.

Maffucci's syndrome

- This syndrome is characterized by the presence of multiple enchondromas and venous malformations.
- The enchondromas are usually found on the hands.

Blue rubber bleb syndrome (Bean syndrome)

- This syndrome is characterized by multiple venous malformations of the:
  - Skin (usually the hands and feet)
  - GI tract.

Proteus syndrome

- This syndrome is named after a Greek god who could change his appearance at will.
- It is characterized by symmetrical overgrowth of bone and soft tissue and development of vascular malformations.

Miscellaneous vascular abnormalities

The following vascular lesions are difficult to classify.

3

Macular stains

- Macular stains are also known as:
  - An angel's kiss
  - A salmon patch
  - A stork mark.
- They occur on the nape of the neck in over 50% of neonates.
- The lesions are flat, pale pink and fade slowly.

Telangiectasia

- Telangiectasia is the presence of visibly dilated vessels within the skin.
- It commonly occurs in the face and legs and can be treated by:
  - Pulse dye laser
  - Injection of sclerosant substances into the dilated vessels.

Pyogenic granuloma

- Pyogenic granulomas may be classified as haemangiomas.
- They are composed of proliferative vascular tissue.
- Pyogenic granulomas grow rapidly and can be confused with malignancies.
- They should be treated with curettage or excision.
- It is important to submit them for histological examination to exclude the presence of malignancy.

Further reading

de Gier HHW, Balm AJM, Bruning PR *et al.* Systematic approach to the treatment of chylous leakage after neck dissection. *Head Neck* 1996; **18** (4): 347–51.

De Mey A, Van Hoof I, De Roy G *et al.* Anatomy of the orbicularis oris muscle in cleft lip. *Br J Plast Surg* 1989; **42** (6): 710–4.

Jackson IT. Classification and treatment of orbitozygomatic and orbitoethmoid fractures. The place of bone grafting and plate fixation. *Clin Plast Surg* 1989; **16** (1): 77–91.

Jones MC. Facial clefting: etiology and developmental pathogenesis. *Clin Plast Surg* 1993; **20** (4): 599–606.

Kohout MP, Hansen M, Pribaz JJ *et al.* Arteriovenous malformations of the head and neck: natural history and management. *Plast Reconstr Surg* 1998; **102** (3): 643–54.

Mulliken JB, Glowacki J. Hemangiomas and vascular malformations in infants and children: a classification based on endothelial characteristics. *Plast Reconstr Surg* 1982; **69** (3): 412–22.

Mulliken JB. Principles and techniques of bilateral complete cleft lip repair. *Plast Reconstr Surg* 1985: **75** (4): 477–87.

Noordhoff MS. Reconstruction of the vermilion in unilateral and bilateral cleft lips. *Plast Reconstr Surg* 1984: **73** (1): 52–61.

O'Brien CJ, Urist MM, Maddox WA. Modified radical neck dissection. Terminology, technique, and indications. *Am J Surg* 1987; **153** (3): 310–6.

Randall P. History of cleft lip nasal repair. *Cleft Palate Craniofac J* 1992; **29** (6): 527–30.

Sassoon EM, Poole MD, Rushworth G. Reanimation for facial palsy using gracilis muscle grafts. *Br J Plast Surg* 1991; **44** (3): 195–200.

Shah JP, Anderson PE. The impact of patterns of nodal metastasis on modifications of neck dissection. *Ann Surg Oncol* 1994; **1** (6): 521–32.

Smith BR, Johnson JV. Rigid fixation of comminuted mandibular fractures. *J Oral Maxillofac Surg* 1993; **51** (12): 1320–6.

Spauwen PH, Goorhuis-Brouwer SM, Schutte HK. Cleft palate repair: Furlow versus von Langenbeck. *J Craniomaxillofac Surg* 1992; **20** (1): 18–20.

Stranc MF, Robertson GA. A classification of injuries to the nasal skeleton. *Ann Plast Surg* 1979; **2** (6): 468–74.

Takenoshita Y, Ishibashi H, Oka M. Comparison of functional recovery after nonsurgical and surgical treatment of condylar fractures. *J Oral Maxillofac Surg* 1990; **48** (11): 1191–5.

Weissman JL, Akindele R. Current imaging techniques for head and neck tumors. *Oncology* 1999; **13** (5): 697–709.

Wells MD, Manktelow RT. Surgical management of facial palsy. *Clin Plast Surg* 1990; **17** (4): 645–53.

Zide BM. Anatomy of the eyelids. *Clin Plast Surg* 1981; **8** (4): 623–34.

4

The breast and chest wall

4

Breast anatomy

- The base of the breast extends vertically from the 2nd to the 6th rib.
- Horizontally it extends from the lateral margin of the sternum to the anterior axillary fold.
- The axillary tail (of Spence) extends upwards and laterally towards the axilla.
- Each breast consists of 15–20 lobes which radiate outwards from the nipple.
- The lobes contain a variable number of lobules.
- Each lobe drains into a mammary duct which terminates on the nipple.
- Most breast cancers originate from mammary ducts.
- Each lobule contains between 10 and 100 acini which drain into the collecting duct.
- The lobes are separated from each other by fibrous septa.
- These septa extend from the skin to the fascia.
- The septa are well developed in the upper portion of the breast, where they are known as the suspensory ligaments of Astley Cooper.

Arterial supply

Blood reaches the breast via the following sources.

- Perforating branches of the internal mammary artery
- Pectoral branches of the thoracoacromial axis
- The lateral thoracic artery
- Lateral branches of the 3rd to 5th intercostal arteries.

Nerve supply

- Breast sensation is provided by the following nerves.
  - The anterior cutaneous branches of the 2nd to 6th intercostal nerves

- The anterior cutaneous branches of the 3rd to 6th lateral cutaneous nerves
- Supraclavicular branches of the cervical plexus.

- The nipple is supplied by branches of the 4th lateral cutaneous nerve.
- One branch of this nerve travels through the breast to the nipple.
- Another traverses medially on the chest wall before ascending vertically towards the nipple.

Surface anatomy

- Penn described a set of ideal breast measurements.
- He found that in an aesthetically pleasing breast:
  1 The sternal notch to nipple distance is roughly equivalent to the distance between the nipples.
  2 On average, this distance is 21 cm.
  3 The distance from the nipple to the inframammary crease is approximately 6.8 cm.
  4 The areolar diameter varies from 3.8 to 4.5 cm.

Breast-cup size

The cup size of a breast is estimated in the following way.

- The chest circumference is measured at the level of the inframammary fold.
- The chest circumference is measured around the most prominent part of the breast.
- The former measurement is subtracted from the latter measurement.
- The difference between the measurements equates to the size of the breast cup.
  - A 4-inch difference: AA cup
  - A 5-inch difference: A cup
  - A 6-inch difference: B cup
  - A 7-inch difference: D cup
  - A 8-inch difference: E cup
  - A 9-inch difference: F cup.

Breast reduction

History

- Thorek described the free-nipple-graft technique of breast reduction in the 1920s.
- Wise described the keyhole pattern of skin incision in the 1950s.
- Strombeck described the horizontal bipedicled technique of breast reduction in 1960.
- Skoog modified Strombeck's design and described the superomedial pedicle technique of breast reduction.
- Mckissock described the vertical bipedicled technique of breast reduction in 1972.
- Weiner described the superior pedicle technique of breast reduction in 1973.

· Ribeiro was the first to describe the inferior pedicle technique of breast reduction in 1975.
· In the last 10 years, Lejour has popularized the vertical scar technique of breast reduction.
· This technique was originally described by Lassus.
· Benelli described the round-block technique of breast reduction in 1990.

Techniques

Techniques of breast reduction can be classified by: (i) the pattern of skin excision; and (ii) variations in the design of the pedicle.

Patterns of skin excision

· The most commonly used pattern of skin excision is the keyhole.
· Regnault has described a skin excision in the shape of a 'B'.
· Lejour has popularized the vertical scar technique of breast reduction.
· Marchac has described a technique with short lateral incisions.
· The periareolar technique has recently been modified and popularised by Benelli.

Design of the pedicle

· In all methods of breast reduction, except the free-nipple-graft technique, it is important to maintain a satisfactory blood supply to the nipple areolar complex (NAC).
· This is achieved by preserving an attachment between the chest wall and the NAC.
· This attachment, or pedicle, may be composed of:
  · Glandular tissue
  · Glandular tissue and de-epithelialized dermis.

Free-nipple-graft technique

· In this technique, the NAC is removed and replaced as a graft.
· The free-nipple-graft technique has the following advantages.
  · It avoids the morbidity associated with maintaining a long pedicle to the NAC.
  · It is relatively quick and easy to perform.
· The free-nipple-graft technique of breast reduction has the following disadvantages.
  · Failure of the NAC to take as a graft can occur.
  · Nipple sensation is lost.
· For these reasons, the use of the free-nipple-graft technique is usually reserved for elderly patients requiring large breast reductions.

Inferior pedicle method

· This is one of the most commonly used techniques of breast reduction.

- This technique has the following advantages.
  - It is relatively simple to learn.
  - It may preserve nipple sensation by maintaining the integrity of the deep branch of the 4th lateral cutaneous nerve.
- The following points are important when using the inferior pedicle technique of breast reduction.

1. The pedicle must remain attached to the chest wall.
   - It is important not to undermine the pedicle.
   - To ensure that it is not undermined, it is important to cut obliquely downwards and outwards when developing the pedicle.
2. The base of the pedicle can be inclined laterally.
   - This increases the chance of the inclusion of sensory branch within the pedicle.
3. In firm breasts, the width of the keyhole pattern should be narrowed.
   - If the pattern is not narrowed, undue tension will be placed on the skin flaps.
   - This can result in their necrosis.
4. The NAC should never be sited too high.
   - A high nipple is extremely difficult to correct.
   - At the end of the procedure, the nipples should lie just below the most prominent part of the breast.

Mastopexy

- Mastopexy is excision of breast skin alone without the underlying gland.
- The technique is used to elevate breasts which have a significant degree of ptosis.
- Ptosis is the natural droop of the breasts.
- Ptosis has been classified by Regnault into the following groups.

First-degree ptosis

The nipples are at, or slightly above, the level of the inframammary fold.

Second-degree ptosis

The nipples lie below the inframammary fold but above the most dependent portion of breast.

Third-degree ptosis

The nipples lie below the inframammary fold and the most dependent portion of breast.

Pseudo-ptosis

- The major portion of the breast mound lies below the inframammary crease.
- The NAC remains at, or slightly above, the level of the inframammary fold.
- This appearance may occur after breast reduction.

Surgical correction of ptosis

The following techniques may be used to correct breast ptosis.

- Augmentation only
  - An implant may be inserted under the breast parenchyma to increase the volume of the breast and improve its contour.
  - This technique can be used to treat minor degrees of ptosis.
  - It is not suitable for more severe ptosis as:
    - An excessively large implant will be required to tighten the slack skin.
    - The ptotic skin may hang over the implant creating an unattractive 'double bubble' or 'snoopy' appearance.
- Circumareolar mastopexy
  - This technique involves de-epithelializing a concentric ring of tissue around the NAC.
  - This skin envelope of the breast is then tightened by suturing the outer margin of the concentric ring to the NAC.
  - Benelli has described a round-block technique of securing the NAC after circumareolar mastopexy, which involves:
    - A purse-string, or round-block, closure of the outer dermal circumference with a permanent suture
    - Insertion of horizontal and vertical sutures through the NAC from one side of the outer dermal circumference to the other.
  - This placement of sutures:
    - Reduces the tendency of the NAC to stretch
    - Reduces the tendency of the NAC and underlying tissues to herniate through the opening maintained by the round-block suture.
- Circumareolar skin excision combined with a vertical or oblique skin excision
  - This technique adds a vertical component to the circumareolar skin excision which:
    - Allows more skin be excised
    - Helps in elevating the NAC.
- Circumareolar skin excision combined with vertical and short horizontal skin excisions
- Circumareolar skin excision combined with a full keyhole-pattern skin excision
  - The full keyhole pattern is used in patient with severe ptosis.
  - This technique permits:
    - Removal of large amounts of excess skin
    - Superior transposition of the NAC into its correct position.

The tuberous breast

- This deformity is also known as a constricted breast.
- It is characterized by the following abnormalities.
  - A deficient breast-base dimension
  - A tight and elevated inframammary fold
  - An elongated thin breast

- Herniation of the NAC
- Stretching of the areola.

Surgical correction

- The tuberous breast is a difficult problem to correct.
- The principles of surgical correction include:
  - Reducing the size of the areola
  - Dividing any constrictions within the breast parenchyma
  - Lowering and releasing the inframammary fold
  - Insertion of an implant or tissue expander.
- Moderate deformities can often be corrected by the insertion of a prosthesis alone.
- More severe deformities are usually treated with a combination of:
  - Release of the constrictions within the breast parenchyma
  - Insertion of a prosthesis or a tissue expander
  - Circumareolar mastopexy
  - The round-block suture technique to limit herniation of the NAC.
- Very severe deformities require importation of extra skin.
- This can be achieved by transposition of a medially based thoraco-epigastric flap from below the inferior mammary crease to the lower medial portion of the breast.

Gynaecomastia

- Gynaecomastia is over-development of the male breast.
- Its incidence varies with age.
  - 75% of boys have some evidence of gynaecomastia at puberty; 75% of these have resolved within 2 years.
  - 7% of 17-year-old boys have significant gynaecomastia.
  - 30% of middle-aged men have significant gynaecomastia.

Causes

The causes of gynaecomastia can be divided into the three ‘P’s.

- **P**hysiological
  - New-born
  - Puberty
  - Old age.
- **P**harmaceutical
  - Cimetidine
  - Digoxin
  - Diazepam
  - Spironolactone
  - Oestrogens.
- **P**athological
  - Cirrhosis

4

- Malnutrition
- Hypogonadism
- Thyroid disease
- Testicular and pituitary tumours.

Classification

Simon classified gynaecomastia into the following groups.

- *Stage 1*: a slight volume increase with no excess skin.
- *Stage 2a*: a moderate volume increase with no excess skin.
- *Stage 2b*: a moderate volume increase with excess skin.
- *Stage 3*: a marked volume increase with excess skin.

Preoperative assessment

Important points in the assessment of patients with gynaecomastia include the following.

History

- Duration of the gynaecomastia
- Presence of pain
- Use of drugs
- Presence of symptoms suggestive of a pathological cause.

Breast examination

- Assessment of the volume of the gynaecomastia
- Estimation of the amount of excess skin present
- Palpation to detect the presence of a firm central core of breast tissue below the NAC
- Palpation for any abnormal breast masses.

General examination

- Examination of the genitalia
- Liver palpation
- Thyroid examination.

Surgical correction

Surgical correction of gynaecomastia may be performed by: (i) liposuction; (ii) excision; or (iii) a combination of liposuction and excision.

Liposuction

- Liposuction alone may be effective in treating mild deformities without a significant central core of breast tissue.
- Liposuction can be used as an adjunct to excisional surgery.
- Recent reports suggest that ultrasonic- and power-assisted liposuction may be better at removing recalcitrant fat deposits.

Excisional techniques

· Excision of the breast tissue can be performed via a semicircular incision along the inferior border of the areola.
· This is known as Webster's operation.
· Access to the breast tissue is relatively poor and it can be difficult to remove the breast tissue completely and evenly.
· Access can be improved by de-epithelializing a doughnut of skin around the NAC.
· The breast tissue is accessed through a transverse incision which passes across the de-epithelialized area.
· The incision deviates below the NAC.
· Following excision of the breast tissue, the skin is closed in a similar fashion to a circumareolar mastopexy.
· Endoscopic resection of breast tissue via a small axillary incision has been reported.

Breast augmentation

· The first breast augmentation with a silicone gel prosthesis was performed by Cronin and Gerow in the early 1960s.
· Since that time, it is now estimated that 1% of women in the USA have undergone breast augmentation.
· Breast augmentation may be classified by: (i) composition of the shell of the implant; (ii) composition of the contents of the implant; (iii) shape of the implant; (iv) incision through which the implant is inserted; and (iv) position into which the implant is inserted.

Composition of the shell

· The shell of most breast implants is composed of silicone.
· The surface of the implant may be:
  · Smooth, or
  · Textured.
· Textured implants are believed to induce less capsular contracture.
· Polyurethane coated implants have been used.
· They had a low rate of capsular contracture.
· Concerns over the formation of toluene by-products, shown to be carcinogenic in animals, resulted in their withdrawal from the market.
· The prophylactic removal of symptom-free, polyurethane-coated implants is not indicated as the risk of surgical removal has been shown to outweigh that of carcinogenesis.

Composition of the contents

The following materials have been used to fill breast implants.

· Liquid silicone gel
· Cohesive silicone gel
· Saline
· Hydrogel

- Triglyceride
- Hyaluronic acid.

Shape

- Breast implants may be:
  - Round, or
  - Shaped.
- Anatomically shaped implants are designed to resemble the contours of the breast.
- They have less projection at their upper border and more projection at their lower border.
- There is some controversy as to whether shaped or round implants produce a better result.
- Proponents of anatomically shaped implants claim that they produce a better breast shape.
- Proponents of non-shaped implants argue:
  - That round implants become shaped when held upright
  - That there is a risk of the shaped implant rotating.

Incisions for insertion

Breast implants can be inserted through the following incisions.

Inframammary incision

- This is probably the most common method of inserting breast implants.
- Advantages include good exposure and ease of pocket dissection.
- Disadvantages include the presence of a visible scar.

Axillary incision

- This incision is hidden in the axilla.
- Dissection of the pocket, particularly medially and inferiorly, may be difficult.
- If this dissection is not completed, the implants tend to displace superiorly.

Periareolar incision

- This approach has the advantage of a concealed scar.
- Nipple paraesthesia and a scar tenderness may occur post-operatively.

Umbilical incision

- Expansion devices can be inserted via the umbilicus to create a cavity under the breast parenchyma.
- Collapsible saline implants are then inserted into the cavity through the small umbilical incision.
- Despite numerous proponents, this approach is not widely practised.

Endoscopic insertion

- The pocket for the breast implant can be dissected endoscopically.
- This reduces the length of the incision.

· This technique is particularly useful for inserting inflatable implants via an umbilical or axillary approach.

Position

Breast implants can be placed in the following locations.

1 A subglandular pocket
- This lies below the breast tissue but superficial to the fascia over the pectoralis major muscle.

2 A subpectoral pocket
- This lies deep to pectoralis major and superficial to pectoralis minor.
- In order to position the implant at the correct height, the inferior pole may lie below the lower border of pectoralis major muscle.
- The inferior border of the implant is therefore not completely covered by muscle.

3 A submuscular pocket
- The bulk of this pocket lies under the pectoralis major muscle.
- Laterally it lies under the serratus anterior muscle.
- Inferiorly it lies under the fascia of the rectus abdominis muscle.

Classification of capsular contraction

- A capsule of connective tissue forms around all implants.
- Baker has classified the degree of capsular contracture into four grades:
  - *Grade 1*: the breast feels soft.
  - *Grade 2*: the capsule around the implant is palpable.
  - *Grade 3*: the capsule around the implant is palpable and visible.
  - *Grade 4*: the capsule around the implant is palpable, visible and painful.
- The exact cause of capsular contracture is unknown but it may result from episodes of subacute infection.

Findings of the Independent Review Group in the UK

- In recent years there has been a great deal of controversy over whether silicone implants are responsible for:
  - Some types of autoimmune disease
  - An increase in the risk of breast cancer
  - Difficulties in screening for cancer.
- An Independent Review Group was set up in the United Kingdom to examine the evidence for these claims.
- In 1998, the report concluded that:
  - Silicone breast implants are not associated with a greater health risk when compared to other surgical implants.
  - There was no evidence of:
    - An association with an abnormal immune response
    - An association with typical or atypical connective tissue diseases or syndromes.
  - Children of implanted women are at no increased risk of connective tissue disease.

- Silicone implants are associated with a number of local complications.
- These local complications include rupture of the implant and the formation of capsules.

- The report recommended the formation of a national implant registry in which the details of all women undergoing breast augmentation are recorded.

Findings of IMNAS in the US

In the United States, the Institute of Medicine of the National Academy of Science (IMNAS) released its final report in June 1999, concluding the following.

- There is no evidence that silicone implants are responsible for any major diseases.
- Women are exposed to silicone constantly in their daily lives.
- There is no evidence that recurrent breast cancer is more prevalent in women with breast implants.
- Silicone breast augmentation is not a contraindication to breast feeding; cows' milk and infant formulas contain a higher level of silica than breast milk from women with silicone implants.

Breast cancer

- Breast cancer is the second most common cancer in women.
- One in 12 women will develop breast cancer in their lifetime.

Risk factors in development

- Breast cancer is associated with early menarche and late menopause.
- A history of maternal breast cancer doubles an individual's risk of developing breast cancer.
- *BRCA 1* is a tumour suppressor gene identified in 1994.
- *BRCA 2* is a tumour suppressor gene identified in 1995.
- All women possess the *BRCA 1* and *2* genes.
- Mutation of these genes inhibits tumour suppression and increases the risk of breast cancer.
- Between one in 200–400 women are carriers of mutations in the *BRCA 1* gene.
- The mutation is inherited in an autosomal dominant manner.
- Women who are carriers of the *BRCA 1* gene mutation have:
  - An 85% lifetime risk of developing breast cancer
  - A 65% chance of developing ovarian cancer by the time they are 70 years of age.
- Mutations of the *BRCA 1* and *2* tumour-supressor genes are estimated to be responsible for 2–3% of all breast cancers.

Pathology

The World Health Organization has classified breast cancers into the following two groups: (i) non-invasive tumours; and (ii) invasive tumours.

- **Non-invasive tumours**
  - Ductal carcinoma *in situ*
    - Ductal carcinoma *in situ* (DCIS) is characterized by dysplasia confined to the epithelial cells of the mammary ducts.
    - It is bilateral in 10% of cases.
    - Multicentric disease within the breast occurs in 20% of cases.
    - 30% of affected patients go on to develop invasive breast cancer.
    - Small lesions are usually treated by local excision.
    - Larger lesions or lesions within smaller breasts are often treated with mastectomy.
  - Lobular carcinoma *in situ*
    - Lobular carcinoma *in situ* (LCIS) is considered a marker, rather than a precursor, of breast cancer.
    - LCIS is bilateral in 40% of cases and multifocal in 60%.
    - Affected patients are estimated to have a 1% chance per year of developing invasive breast cancer.
    - Some affected patients opt to undergo bilateral prophylactic mastectomy to reduce the risk of developing invasive disease.
- **Invasive tumours**
  - Invasive ductal carcinoma
  - Invasive lobular carcinoma
  - Medullary carcinoma
  - Tubular carcinoma
  - Papillary carcinoma
  - Mucinous carcinoma
  - Adenoid cystic carcinoma.
- Ductal carcinoma is responsible for 75% of invasive tumours.
- Lobular carcinoma is responsible for 10% of invasive tumours.

The TNM classification

- T*is*: *in situ* carcinoma
- T1: a tumour <2 cm in diameter
- T2: a tumour 2–5 cm in diameter
- T3: a tumour >5 cm in diameter
- T4: a tumour that invades the skin or chest wall
- N1: ipsilateral mobile lymphadenopathy
- N2: ipsilateral fixed lymphadenopathy
- N3: involvement of the internal mammary nodes
- M0: no distant metastases
- M1: supraclavicular nodes or distant metastases.

Staging

- *Stage 0*: T*is* N0 M0
- *Stage 1*: T1 N0 M0

- *Stage 2a*: T1 N1 M0, T2 N0 M0
- *Stage 2b*: T2 N1 M0, T3 N0 M0
- *Stage 3a*: T0 N2 M0, T1 N2 M0, T2 N2 M0, T3 N1 M0, T3 N2 M0
- *Stage 3b*: T4 any N any M, any T N3
- *Stage 4*: any T any N M1.

Survival rates

According to the American Joint Committee on Cancer Staging (AJCCS), breast cancer is associated with the following 5-year survival rates for each stage.

- *Stage 1*: 85%
- *Stage 2*: 66%
- *Stage 3*: 41%
- *Stage 4*: 10%.

Biological behaviour

- 80% of breast cancers are adenocarcinomas.
- 50% of all malignant tumours occur in the upper half of the breast.
- The risk of distant metastases increases proportionately with the number of positive axillary nodes.
- Metastases tend to occur in the following sites.
  - Lung
  - Liver
  - Bone.

Mammography

- In the United Kingdom, the national screening program involves mammography every 2–3 years for women between 50 and 65 years of age.
- The American Cancer Society recommends annual mammography for women over 40 years of age.
- The benefit of routine screening of patients between 40 and 50 years of age is controversial.
- Patients with a strong family history should have earlier mammography.
- The diagnostic value of mammography is limited in the younger patient.
- The increased fibrous nature of the breast of young patients makes the detection of abnormalities more difficult.
- Ultrasound is useful particularly in the younger patient to differentiate between solid and cystic lesions.
- Suspicious signs on mammography include:
  - Microcalcification
  - Density changes
  - Asymmetry
  - Architectural distortion.
- Swedish trials have demonstrated a 44% decrease in mortality from breast cancer in patients undergoing regular mammography.

Surgical treatment

Primary tumours

The primary tumour may be excised in the following ways.

Lumpectomy

- This form of treatment is primarily indicated for patients with stage 1 and 2 disease.
- It is not suitable for:
  - Patients with widespread disease
  - Patients with small breasts.
- Lumpectomy is usually followed by radiotherapy directed at the site of the primary tumour.

Quadrantectomy

- This operation aims to remove an entire quadrant of the breast.
- It is primarily used to treat T2 tumours.
- A significant deformity may result if the defect is not reconstructed.

Subcutaneous mastectomy

- In this procedure, 90–95% of the breast tissue is removed.
- The NAC is preserved.
- When used prophylactically, it is a cancer-reducing rather than cancer-preventing procedure as some breast tissue remains.
- There have been reports of breast cancer occurring in patients who have previously had a subcutaneous mastectomy.
  - Immediate reconstruction is usually performed following subcutaneous mastectomy by either:
    - An implant or expander placed in a submuscular position, or
    - A de-epithelialized transverse rectus abdominis muscle (TRAM) flap.

Total (simple) mastectomy

- Total mastectomy is usually performed in:
  - Stage 3 or 4 disease
  - Stage 2 disease in patients with small breasts.

The axilla

- The axilla may be treated by:
  - Axillary clearance
  - Biopsy followed by post-operative radiotherapy if the nodes are positive.
- During axillary clearance, the following levels can be removed.
  - *Level 1*: this lies below and lateral to the pectoralis minor muscle
  - *Level 2*: this lies behind the pectoralis minor muscle
  - *Level 3*: this lies above and medial to pectoralis minor muscle.
- In a Halsted mastectomy, the pectoralis major and minor muscles are excised.

- Axillary sampling involves removal of the contents of part of level 1.
- Adequate axillary sampling requires the inclusion of at least five lymph nodes.
- Sentinel node biopsy has recently been used to stage the axilla.
- This technique aims to identify the first (sentinel) node to which the tumour drains.
- Histological sampling of this node:
  - Is believed to accurately stage the axilla
  - Avoids the morbidity associated with a traditional axillary clearance.

Adjuvant therapy

- Post-operative radiotherapy is given to patients undergoing lumpectomy for invasive carcinoma.
- Post-operative chemotherapy appears to prolong the disease-free survival in pre-menopausal women.
- The benefit of chemotherapy in post-menopausal women is unclear.
- The 'CMF' chemotherapy regimen is often used.
- This consists of:
  - **C**yclophosphamide
  - **M**ethotrexate
  - 5 **F**luouracil.
- Tamoxifen is known to be beneficial for post-menopausal women.
- In recent years, tamoxifen has also been shown to have a beneficial effect on survival in premenopausal women.

Breast reconstruction

- With increased patient awareness and the wider availability of genetic screening, an increasing number of women are seeking breast reconstruction.
- Breast reconstruction may be:
  1. Performed at the time of tumour excision (immediate reconstruction)
  2. Performed at a later date (delayed reconstruction).
- The available methods of breast reconstruction include:
  - Oncoplastic techniques
  - Insertion of a breast implant or expander
  - Insertion of a breast implant or expander combined with flap reconstruction
  - Flap reconstruction alone.

Oncoplastic surgery

- This is a relatively new technique which involves tumour-specific immediate breast reconstruction.
- Breast conservation surgery, particularly lower-pole quadrantectomies, can result in significant deformities.
- Using techniques developed during breast reduction and mastopexy surgery, these defects can be reconstructed primarily at the time of the ablative surgery.

- Lesions in the lower quadrants of large breasts can be reconstructed by:
  - Excision of the tumour as part of the tissue removed during a breast reduction
  - Reconstruction of the breast in a similar fashion to a superior pedicle keyhole pattern breast reduction
  - Reduction of the contralateral breast in a similar fashion to maintain symmetry.
- Medial lesions in large breasts can be reconstructed by:
  - Excision of the tumour as part of the tissue removed during a keyhole pattern breast reduction
  - Reconstruction of the medial defect with a dermoglandular flap based on the lateral limb of the vertical part of the keyhole incision.
- Central upper pole lesions can be reconstructed by:
  - Excision of the tumour using an upside-down keyhole pattern
  - Reconstruction of the resultant defect in the shape of a 'T'.
- In patients with large breasts, it is usually possible to excise the tumour and, rather than directly close the defect, reconstruct it with local tissue.

Inserting implants or expanders

- This technique work best in small breasts (A or B cup).
- It requires the presence of healthy non-irradiated overlying skin.
- Reconstruction can be performed with:
  - Simple implants
  - Tissue expanders.
- Tissue expanders have the advantages of:
  - Being adjustable
  - Creating some degree of ptosis if they are initially over-expanded and then partially deflated.
- Round implants or expanders work best in women with small round breasts.
- Shaped implants or expanders are often used to reconstruct larger breasts with more projection.
- The base position and the dimensions of the prosthesis should be matched to the contralateral side.
- The base of the implant or expander should be placed at, or slightly lower, than the level of the contralateral inframammary fold.
- The implant should be placed under the pectoralis major muscle whenever possible.
- The inframammary fold can be reconstructed by suturing subcutaneous tissue to the underlying fascia at the required level.

Tissue expanders available for breast reconstruction include the following.

The Becker expander

- The outer lumen of these expanders is filled with low-bleed silicone gel.
- The inner lumen is expandable and is filled with saline.
- The implants are available with a smooth or textured shell.
- The silicone gel accounts for approximately 25% of the volume of the implant when expanded.

· Expansion is performed though a remote port.
· When expansion is completed, the remote port is removed from the expander by traction.
· The contents of the expander are retained by a self-sealing valve.
· The expander may be replaced with a fixed-volume implant once the desired breast size and shape is achieved.

The McGhan biodimensional expander
· This is a shaped implant with more projection inferiorly.
· The implant has a textured shell and is available in varying shapes and dimensions.
· Expansion is performed through an integral magnetic valve in the upper portion of the shell.
· The valve is located with a magnet prior to expansion.

Inserting implants or expanders combined with flap reconstruction

· This type of reconstruction is usually performed with an implant placed underneath a transposed latissimus dorsi musculocutaneous flap.
· The indications for this type of reconstruction include:
  · Cases unsuitable for reconstruction with an implant alone.
  · Cases where autologous-only reconstruction is not appropriate.
· This method of breast reconstruction has the following advantages:
  · It is relatively easy to perform.
  · The flap is reliable.
  · It places well-vascularized tissue over the implant.
  · It is associated with a low complication rate.
· The technique has the following disadvantages:
  · A prosthesis, with all its inherent risks, is required.
  · It leaves an unsightly donor site on the back.

Flap reconstruction alone

Breast reconstruction with flaps can be performed by: (i) pedicled transfers; and (ii) free transfers.

Pedicled transfers
Pedicled transfers commonly used for breast reconstruction include the following.

The latissimus dorsi flap
· The traditional latissimus dorsi flap does not usually provide sufficient tissue for autologous-only reconstruction.
· Extended latissimus dorsi flaps have been described.
· These include subcutaneous tissue peripheral to the skin flap.
· This design is particularly useful in women with significant amounts of subcutaneous tissue.

- Variations in the design of the skin paddle have been described, including:
  - Crescentic flaps
  - Trefoil flaps.
- The trefoil flap is composed of a horizontal skin paddle with a vertical V-shaped extension extending superiorly towards the axilla.

Pedicled-TRAM flaps

- The blood supply of the pedicled-TRAM flap is from the superior epigastric vessels.
- The flap can be based on one, or both, rectus abdominis muscles.
- Some authorities advocate complete detachment of the upper end of the muscle from the ribcage to facilitate easy transposition.
- Delaying the flap by dividing the dominant deep inferior epigastric vessels as a primary procedure may improve flap survival.
- Supercharging or turbocharging the flap by anastomosing the deep inferior epigastric artery (DIEA) to the thoracodorsal axis has been suggested as a means of increasing flap perfusion.
- Breast reconstruction with a pedicled-TRAM flap has the following advantages.
  - It is relatively simple and quick to perform.
  - It avoids the need for an implant.
- Breast reconstruction with a pedicled-TRAM flap has the following disadvantages.
  - It produces significant donor site morbidity particularly if both recti muscles are harvested.
  - It may produce an unsightly bulge in the hypogastric region.
  - The flap may be difficult to shape and accurately position due to limitations imposed by the pedicle.
  - It has a high rate of local complications (particularly fat necrosis) when compared to the better perfused free-TRAM flap.

Free-tissue transfers

Free-tissue transfers commonly used for breast reconstruction include the following.

The free-TRAM flap

- This is probably the autologous flap of choice for breast reconstruction.
- It is not suitable for patients who have previously had:
  - Abdominal liposuction
  - Abdominoplasty
  - Midline abdominal incisions.
- The skin paddle is usually based on the contralateral rectus abdominis muscle if branches of the thoracodorsal axis are to be used as the donor vessels.
- The skin paddle is usually based on the ipsilateral rectus abdominis muscle if the internal mammary artery and vein are to be used as the donor vessels.
- The skin paddle of the TRAM flap is divided into four zones.
  - Zone 1 lies over the rectus abdominis muscle.
  - Zone 4 lies on the opposite side of the abdomen in the territory supplied by the contralateral superficial circumflex iliac artery (SCIA).

- There is some confusion over differentiation of zones 2 and 3; different authors interchange these areas.
- Zone 1 lies over the perforators from the DIEA.
- Blood to zone 4 has to travel through two sets of choke vessels from the contralateral DIEA.
- Consequently, zone 4 is relatively poorly perfused and is usually discarded.
- Perforating vessels passing through the rectus muscle from the DIEA are usually located along two rows situated medially and laterally.
- The lateral perforators are dominant in 55% of patients.
- The medial perforators are dominant in 18% of patients.
- A single row of medial perforators is present in 27% of patients.
- The majority of the perforators from the DIEA are centred around the umbilicus.
- The TRAM flap should include these perforators.
- The whole width of the rectus abdominis muscle does not need to be harvested with the flap.
- Removal of a minimal amount of the rectus abdominis muscle and the anterior rectus sheath limits the abdominal morbidity associated with TRAM flap harvest.
- It is important to include the internal oblique muscle in the closure of the rectus sheath.
- This helps prevent post-operative abdominal bulging.

Deep inferior epigastric perforator flaps

- The deep inferior epigastric perforator (DIEP) flap procedure reconstructs the breast with the same skin and soft-tissue paddle as the TRAM flap.
- However, the flap is based on one or two perforators from the DIEA.
- The perforators are preserved by careful intramuscular dissection.
- During dissection the motor nerve fibres supplying the rectus abdominis muscle are preserved as they traverse horizontally through the muscle.
- The DIEA is ligated distally and gently pulled through the split in the rectus abdominis muscle.
- This method of breast reconstruction has the following advantages.
  - It results in less donor site morbidity as the function of the rectus abdominis muscle is preserved.
  - A greater length of pedicle is available.
- This method of breast reconstruction has the following disadvantages.
  - It is technically difficult to perform.
  - It lengthens the time required for flap harvest.
  - It may be associated with a higher rate of flap complications, particularly fat necrosis.

Superior gluteal flaps

- In this technique, the breast is reconstructed with tissue based over the superior gluteal vessels.
- The limited length of available pedicle hinders the routine use of this flap.

Superior gluteal perforator flaps

- During superior gluteal perforator (S-GAP) flap harvest, a perforating vessel is isolated and dissected through the gluteus maximus muscle proximally to the superior gluteal artery.
- Up to 5–8 cm of pedicle is available.
- The pedicle is longer than that of the conventional superior gluteal flap as it includes the length of the intramuscular portion of the perforator.
- Skin paddles of up to 29 × 3 cm are available.
- Closure of the excised defect acts as a unilateral thigh lift.

Rubens flaps

- This flap reconstructs the breast with the soft-tissue pad overlying the iliac crest.
- This soft-tissue pad was apparently particularly prominent in ladies painted by Rubens.
- The flap is based on the deep circumflex iliac vessels.
- It is important to accurately repair the muscles at the donor site following flap harvest.
- This flap is usually used for patients in which other autologous options are not available.

Reconstructing the NAC

- Reconstruction of the NAC is usually performed at least 3 months after breast reconstruction.
- This is because it is difficult to correctly site the NAC at the time of breast reconstruction.
- Before NAC reconstruction, the patient is asked to decide on the placement of the NAC.
- They do this by placing an adhesive ECG electrode at the desired NAC position.
- Reconstruction of the NAC involves:
  - Reconstruction of the nipple
  - Reconstruction of the areola.

Nipple reconstruction

This is usually performed by one of the following techniques.

Nipple sharing

In this procedure, the nipple is reconstructed with a portion of the contralateral nipple used as a composite graft.

Skate flap

- In this procedure, the nipple is reconstructed with a local flap which is said to resemble a skate fish.
- This technique leaves a de-epithelialized donor site around its periphery.
- A full-thickness skin graft is applied to this area to reconstruct the areola.

Star flap

- This is a modification of the skate flap.
- It allows direct closure of the lateral donor sites.
- The areola is then reconstructed by tattooing.

Tripod or quadripod flaps

- These techniques involve elevating flaps shaped like three- and four-bladed propellers.
- The centre of the flap is drawn up and the blades of the propeller are used to reconstruct the sides of the nipple.
- This technique is subject to retraction post-operatively.

4

Other methods

- The double-opposing tab (DOT) flap
- The C-V flap.

Areola reconstruction

This is usually performed by one of the following techniques.

Full-thickness skin graft

- This may be obtained from the contralateral areola if the patient is undergoing simultaneous contralateral breast reduction or mastopexy.
- Alternatively, it can be obtained from the non-hairy skin lateral to the labia majora.
- This area is chosen because the pigmentation of grafts taken from this site matches that of the areola.

Tattooing

- Areolar tattooing can be performed at the time of nipple reconstruction or at a later date.
- The colour of the tattoo tends to fade with time.
- If this occurs, tattooing may need to be repeated.

Chest wall reconstruction

Embryology and anatomy

- The ribs, costal cartilages and sternum begin to develop at the 6th week of gestation.
- The sternum arises from paired mesodermal bands.
- These fuse at the 9th week of gestation.
- The 1st–7th ribs fuse with the sternum at the 9th week of gestation.
- Inspiratory muscles pull the ribcage upwards.
- Inspiratory muscles include:
  - The sternocleidomastoid muscle
  - The scalene muscles.

- Expiratory muscles pull the ribcage downwards.
- Expiratory muscles include:
  - The rectus abdominis muscle
  - The external oblique muscle
  - The internal oblique muscle.
- A flail segment moves paradoxically with breathing and requires stabilization and reconstruction.
- A flail segment results after excision of:
  - More than four neighbouring ribs
  - >5 cm of the chest wall.

Pectus deformities

- Pectus deformities occur once in approximately every 300 live births.
- Pectus excavatum (a concave chest) is the most common deformity.
- Pectus carinatum (a convex or pigeon chest) is less common.

Pectus excavatum

- This occurs as a result of abnormal growth of the costal cartilages.
- The sternum is displaced posteriorly and in severe cases can lie in contact with the vertebral bodies.
- Pectus excavatum can be corrected by:
  - The insertion of a prosthetic moulage
  - Reconstruction of the ribcage.
- The ribcage can be reconstructed with the Ravitch procedure.
- This involves:
  1. Elevation of perichondrial flaps from the costal cartilages
  2. Resection of the abnormal costal cartilages with preservation of the costo-chondral junction
  3. Osteotomies of the upper and lower parts of the sternum which is then mobilized anteriorly
  4. Stabilization of the sternum in its new position with wires or bars
  5. Suture of the pectoralis muscles over the sternum in the midline.
- An alternative method of correcting pectus excavatum involves:
  1. Complete mobilization and removal of the sternum
  2. Turning over and shaping the sternum with anterior osteotomies
  3. Replacing and stabilizing the sternum.

Poland's syndrome

- This syndrome was first described by Alfred Poland in 1841 while he was an anatomy demonstrator at Guy's Hospital in London.
- It is a relatively common abnormality.
- It is more common in males but more females request reconstruction.
- It is more common on the right side.
- Poland's syndrome is thought to be caused by kinking of the subclavian artery at around the 6th week of gestation.

- The syndrome is characterized by unilateral chest-wall and upper-limb abnormalities.
- The manifestation of the syndrome is variable and ranges from very mild to severe deformities.

The chest wall

Chest wall deformities associated with Poland's syndrome include:

- Absence of the sternal head of the pectoralis major muscle
- Hypoplasia of the breast and the NAC
- Lack of axillary hair
- Abnormalities of the pectoralis minor muscle, latissimus dorsi muscle, serratus anterior muscle and rectus abdominis muscles.

Upper limb deformities

Upper limb deformities associated with Poland's syndrome include:

- Short arms
- The presence of short, fused fingers (symbrachydactyly); symbrachydactyly is usually limited to the central three digits.

Surgical correction

The following techniques have been used to correct deformities associated with Poland's syndrome.

- Reconstruction of the underlying chest wall deformity
- Reconstruction of the breast mound with an implant or tissue expander
- Reconstruction of the breast mound with an implant or tissue expander combined with a flap
- Flap reconstruction, usually performed with one of the following:
  - A latissimus dorsi flap
  - A TRAM flap.

Sternal dehiscence

- Sternal dehiscence occurs after approximately 1% of median sternotomies.
- Its incidence is increased if one, or both, internal mammary arteries are harvested for coronary artery bypass grafts.
- Sternal dehiscence has been classified by Pairolero.
  - *Type 1*: characterized by a serosanguinous discharge without any evidence of cellulitis, costochondritis or osteomyelitis
  - *Type 2*: characterized by a purulent mediastinitis associated with costochondritis and osteomyelitis
  - *Type 3*: characterized by chronic wound infection associated with costochondritis and osteomyelitis.
- Reconstruction involves excision of all necrotic and non-viable tissue.
- This tissue should be submitted for microbiological analysis.
- The resultant dead space must be filled with well-vascularized tissue from one of the following sources.

Pectoralis major muscle flap

The pectoralis major muscle can be used as a:

- Turnover flap based on its medial perforators
- Transposition flap based on the pectoral branches of the thoraco-acromial axis.

Rectus abdominis muscle flap

- The rectus abdominis muscle can be used as:
  - A muscle-only flap
  - A muscle-and-skin flap
- If the skin paddle is orientated vertically, the flap is known as a vertical rectus abdominis muscle (VRAM) flap.
- This flap receives its blood supply from the superior epigastric artery.
- The superior epigastric artery is a branch of the internal mammary artery.
- This flap should be used with caution in cases in which the internal mammary vessels have been harvested for coronary grafts.
- After harvesting of the internal mammary vessels, muscle perfusion may be maintained from the 8th intercostal artery.

Omental flap

- An omental flap, based on either of the gastro-epiploic pedicles, can be transposed to fill a sternal defect.
- The flap is subsequently skin grafted.

Further reading

Arnold PG, Pairolero PC. Chest wall reconstruction: an account of 500 consecutive cases. *Plast Reconstr Surg* 1996; **98** (5): 804–10.

Barton FE, English JM, Kingsley WB *et al.* Glandular excision in total glandular mastectomy and modified radical mastectomy: a comparison. *Plast Reconstr Surg* 1991; **88** (3): 389–92.

Benelli L. A new periareolar mammaplasty: the 'round block' technique. *Aesthetic Plast Surg* 1990; **14** (2): 93–100.

Blackburn WD, Everson MP. Silicone-associated rheumatic disease: an unsupported myth. *Plast Reconstr Surg* 1997; **99** (5): 1362–7.

Brody GS. On the safety of breast implants. *Plast Reconstr Surg* 1997; **100** (5): 1314–21.

Cohen BE, Biggs TM, Cronin ED *et al.* Assessment and longevity of the silicone gel implant. *Plast Reconstr Surg* 1997; **99** (6): 1597–601.

Dinner MI, Dowden RV. The tubular/tuberous breast syndrome. *Ann Plast Surg* 1987; **19** (5): 414–20.

Dowden RV. Selection criteria for successful immediate breast reconstruction. *Plast Reconstr Surg* 1991; **88** (4): 628–34.

Elliot LF, Eskenazi L, Beegle PH *et al.* Immediate TRAM flap breast reconstruction: 128 consecutive cases. *Plast Reconstr Surg* 1993; **92** (2): 217–27.

Hang-Fu L. Subjective comparison of six different reduction mammaplasty procedures. *Aesthetic Plast Surg* 1991; **15** (4): 297–302.

Hester TR, Bostwick J. Poland's syndrome: correction with latissimus dorsi muscle transposition. *Plast Reconstr Surg* 1982; **69** (2): 226–33.

Lassus C. A 30-year experience with vertical mammaplasty. *Plast Reconstr Surg* 1996; **97** (2): 373–80.

Lejour M. Vertical mammaplasty and liposuction of the breast. *Plast Reconstr Surg* 1994; **94** (1): 100–14.

Malata CM, Feldberg L, Beegle PH *et al.* Textured or smooth implants for breast augmentation? Three year follow-up of a prospective randomised controlled trial. *Br J Plast Surg* 1997; **50** (2): 99–105.

McCraw JP, Papp C, Edwards A *et al.* The autogenous latissimus breast reconstruction. *Clin Plast Surg* 1994; **21** (2): 279–88.

Regnault P. Breast ptosis. Definition and treatment. *Clin Plast Surg* 1976; **3** (2):193–203.

Robbins TH. A reduction mammaplasty with the areola-nipple based on an inferior dermal pedicle. *Plast Reconstr Surg* 1977; **59** (1): 64–7.

Sarhadi NS, Shaw Dunn J, Lee FD *et al.* An anatomical study of the nerve supply of the breast, including the nipple and areola. *Br J Plast Surg* 1996; **49** (3): 156–64.

Warmuth MA, Sutton LM, Winer EP. A review of hereditary breast cancer: from screening to risk factor modification. *Am J Med* 1997; **102** (4): 407–15.

5

The upper limb

Embryology

Developmental anatomy

- The upper limb is derived from lateral plate mesoderm located in the flank of the developing embryo.
- The limb bud first appears on the 26th day of gestation.
- Initially, it consists of a core of proliferating mesenchymal cells covered by an epithelial layer.
- This layer thickens at the tip of the bud in the anteroposterior (AP) axis to form the apical ectodermal ridge (AER).
- Spinal nerves begin to grow into the limb bud a few days after it first appears.
- The limb bud is initially supplied by a capillary network.
- This soon coalesces into a main stem artery which drains into a marginal vein.
- By the 33rd day of gestation, a paddle-shaped hand is present.
- Prechondrogenic condensations of mesenchyme develop at the sites where the cartilagenous skeletal elements will form.
- By the 36th day of gestation, overt chondrogenesis is in progress.
- Myoblasts migrate into the limb and aggregate into two muscle masses—one ventral and one dorsal.
- By the 42nd day of gestation, digital rays are present and the hand assumes a webbed appearance.
- During the 7th week of gestation, the upper limbs rotate 90° laterally to bring the palm anteriorly.
- At the same time, the elbow begins to flex.
- During this period, ossification begins and digital separation occurs.
- Involution of the tissue between the finger rays occurs by programmed cell death (apoptosis).

· By the 8th week of gestation, the upper extremity resembles a miniature adult upper limb.

Mechanisms of development

· Most of the work on the mechanism of limb development has involved moving and transplanting areas of tissue within the chick embryo.
· Recently, some of the molecules involved in limb development have been identified.
· Three main sets of cell interactions are integral to limb development; they include:

1 AER–mesenchmal interactions
  · These are required for bud outgrowth.
  · Resection of the AER results in a truncated limb.
  · Grafting of the AER can extend the limbs of chick embryos.
2 Epithelial–mesenchyme interactions
  · These interactions appear to control the dorsoventral development of the limb.
  · If a segment of right ectoderm is transplanted onto a left limb, a right hand develops.
3 Mesenchymal–mesenchymal interactions
  · These occur between the polarizing region (posterior limb bud mesenchyme) and the limb bud tip mesenchyme.
  · These interactions appear to control the axial development of the limb.
  · If a polarizing region is grafted anteriorly, a mirror set of digits results.

Molecular biology of development

· The function of the AER can be replicated by fibroblast growth factors (FGFs).
· Beads containing FGF2, 4 and 8 can induce normal limb development if the AER has been removed.
· The gene *Wnt-7a* is located in the dorsal regions of the ectodermal tip and is thought to play a role in the dorsoventral orientation of the limb.
· Both retinoic acid (RA) and the product of the sonic hedgehog gene have been shown to mimic the role of the polarizing zone.
· The posterior part of the limb bud contains the highest concentration of RA.
· The subsequent AP concentration gradient is believed to be important in determining the pattern of digital development.
· *Hox d* genes are important in limb patterning.
· Mutations in *Hox d13* are associated with central polydactyly in humans.
· *Gli 3* is another gene involved in the complex molecular pattern of limb development.
· Mutations in this gene cause a variety of polydactylies in humans.

Congenital deformities

Classification

The American Society of Hand Surgery recommends the following classification of congenital hand deformities.

1 *Failure of formation*
- Transverse arrest
  - Complete deficiencies
  - Intercalated deficiencies
- Longitudinal arrest
  - Preaxial—radial club hand
  - Central—central ray deficiency
  - Post-axial—ulnar club hand.

2 *Failure of differentiation*
- Soft tissue
  - Syndactyly
  - Camptodactyly
  - Trigger thumb
  - Clasped thumb
- Skeletal
  - Clinodactyly
  - Symphalangism
  - Synostosis
  - Arthrogryposis
  - Windblown hand.

3 *Duplication*
- Ulnar polydactyly
- Central polydactyly
- Radial polydactyly
- Ulnar dimelia.

4 *Overgrowth*
- Macrodactyly.

5 *Undergrowth*
- Brachydactyly
- Thumb hypoplasia.

6 *Constriction ring syndromes*
- Groups 1–4.

7 *Generalized skeletal abnormalities*

Failure of formation

Transverse

Complete

- This can occur at any level.
- It is most common at the junction of the proximal third and the middle-third of the forearm.
- Treatment is usually non-surgical and involves the fitting of a suitable prosthesis.

Intercalated

- Phocomelia is an intercalated deficiency of the upper limb.
- It occurred with a high incidence in the 1960s as a result of the use of the anti-emetic thalidomide.
- Thalidomide is still used in certain parts of the world as a treatment for leprosy.
- Phocomelia has been subdivided into three categories.
  1 Complete phocomelia—the hand is directly attached to the torso
  2 Proximal phocomelia—the normal forearm and hand are attached to the torso
  3 Distal phocomelia—the hand is attached to the upper arm at the elbow.

Longitudinal

Radial club hand

- This is the most common of the longitudinal deficiencies.
- It occurs with an incidence of between one in 30 000 and one in 100 000 live births.

5

Associated abnormalities

- Radial club hand is associated with a number of cardiovascular, gastro-intestinal, renal and haematological abnormalities.
- Syndromes associated with radial club hand include:
  - Holt–Oram syndrome
    - Radial club hand and cardiac abnormalities
  - VATERR syndrome
    - **V**ertebral anomalies, **a**nal atresia, **t**racheo**e**sphageal fistula and **r**enal and **r**adial abnormalities
  - TAR syndrome
    - **T**hrombocytopaenia and **a**bsent **r**adius
  - Fanconi's anaemia
    - Radial club hand and aplastic anaemia.

Clinical features

The clinical features of radial club hand include:

- A short forearm which is bowed on the radial side
- Complete or partial absence of the radius which is replaced by a fibrous band (anlage)
- A radially deviated hand
- Skin deficiency on the radial side with relative excess on the ulnar side
- A hypoplastic or absent thumb
- Flexion contracture and stiffness of the fingers
- Stiffness of the elbow which may or may not be due to bony fusion (synostosis)
- Hypoplasia or absence of radial structures including the trapezium, scaphoid, 1st metacarpal, radial artery, superficial branch of the radial nerve and radial-sided musculature.

Classification

Radial club hand has been subcategorized into four types.

- *Type 1*: short distal radius
- *Type 2*: hypoplastic radius
- *Type 3*: partial absence of the radius
- *Type 4*: total absence of the radius.

Treatment

- Treatment is based on the patient's age, the severity of the deformity and the degree of functional deficit.
- Surgery is usually performed at approximately 6 months of age.
- Treatment may consist of the following:
  - Splintage and manipulation
    - Physiotherapy to the elbow is particularly important to prevent the progression of stiffness which can result in difficulty with everyday tasks such as eating.
  - Centralization
    - The hand is repositioned over the ulna and stabilized with pin fixation through the 3rd metacarpal.
    - A Z-plasty may be required to release the soft-tissue deficiency on the radial side of the wrist.
    - Some authors recommend including the redundant skin on the ulnar side of the wrist as a transposition flap to release the radial contracture.
  - Radialization
    - The scaphoid is placed over the ulna and secured with pin fixation through the 2nd metacarpal.
    - Transfer of the flexor carpi radialis (FCR) and ulnaris tendons to the ulnar side of the carpus or the 5th metacarpal may help to decrease the radially deforming force.
  - Pollicization of the index finger
    - This procedure is indicated in cases with a severely hypoplastic thumb.
    - Pollicization aims to reproduce the function of the thumb by shortening and rotating the index finger.
    - Pollicization is performed by:

    1 Elevating a dorsal flap from the radial side of the index finger.
    2 Transposing this flap to create the first web space.
    3 Preserving the digital vessels which will supply the transposed index finger.
    4 Performing interfascicular dissection on the common digital nerve to the index finger–middle finger web.
    5 Removing the index metacarpal except for its head which will act as the new trapezium.
    6 Resecting the metacarpal epiphysis to prevent subsequent metacarpal growth.
    7 Rotating the metacarpal head 160°; this will subsequently relax to approximately 120° which is ideal for opposition.

8 Securing the remaining metacarpal head in 40° of palmar abduction.

9 Securing the metacarpal in mild flexion, as the metacarpophalangeal joint of the index finger can hyperextend while that of the joint it aims to replicate (the carpometacarpal joint (CMCJ) of the thumb) does not.

10 Shortening the extensor tendons but not the flexors as the latter take up the slack produced by removing the metacarpal.

11 Repositioning the muscle attachments so that:

- The extensor indicis proprius (EIP) acts as the extensor pollicis longus (EPL).
- The extensor digitorum communis (EDC) to the index finger acts as the abductor pollicis longus (APL).
- The 1st palmar interosseous acts as the abductor pollicis.
- The 1st dorsal interosseous muscle acts as the abductor pollicis brevis (APB) muscle.

Central ray deficiency

5

- This deformity is also known as 'typical cleft hand'.
- It is characterized by partial or complete absence of the central ray (middle finger in the hand, 3rd toe in the foot).
- It is often bilateral and commonly involves both hands and feet.
- A positive family history is common.
- 'Atypical cleft hand' is an old term for a condition now known as 'symbrachydactyly'.
- Symbrachydactyly is characterized by the presence of short vestigial digits which look like small nubbins and often include a vestigial nail.
- Symbrachydactyly in contrast to central ray deficiency:
  - Is usually unilateral
  - Seldom involves the feet
  - Is not usually associated with a positive family history
  - Is classified as a failure of differentiation.

Treatment

- Patients often have remarkably good hand function, and the condition has been labelled as a functional triumph but a social disaster.
- Surgical techniques involve closure of the cleft directly with reapproximation of the metacarpals by reconstruction of the transverse metacarpal ligament.
- The Snow–Littler technique involves raising a dorsal flap from the cleft and transposing it radially to the first web.
- The 2nd metacarpal is then transferred to the 3rd metacarpal base.

Ulnar club hand

- This condition is one-tenth as common as its preaxial counterpart, radial club hand.
- A broad spectrum of abnormalities can occur, ranging from slight hypoplasia of the ulnar digits to total absence of the ulna.

- Ulnar club hand differs from radial club hand in a number of ways.
  - The hand is stable at the wrist but unstable at the elbow. This contrasts with radial club hand in which the wrist is unstable but the elbow is stable or stiff.
  - While radial deficiencies are associated with cardiovascular, haematological and gastro-intestinal abnormalities, ulnar club hand is associated with abnormalities of the musculoskeletal system.
  - In radial club hand, the radius is most commonly totally absent. In ulnar club hand, partial absence of the ulna is the most common finding.

Classification

Ulnar club hand has been classified into four types:

- *Type 1*: hypoplasia of the ulna
- *Type 2*: partial absence of the ulna
- *Type 3*: total absence of the ulna with a normal radiohumoral joint
- *Type 4*: fusion of the radius to the humerus with no elbow joint (radiohumoral synostosis).

Treatment

- Treatment depends on the severity of the deformity.
- Surgical treatment involves release of the fibrous anlage and realignment of the carpus and forearm.

Failure of differentiation

Soft-tissue failures of differentiation

Syndactyly

- The term is derived from the Greek, 'syn' meaning 'together' and 'dactylos' meaning 'digit'.
- Syndactyly is thought to arise as a result of failure of programmed cell death (apoptosis) in interdigital tissue.

Epidemiology

- Syndactyly occurs approximately once in every 1000 and 3000 live births.
- 20% of cases have a positive family history and 30% are bilateral.
- Syndactyly is twice as common in males.
- It is common in Caucasian races.
- Syndactyly may be associated with other congenital deformities such as Apert's and Poland's syndrome.

Classification

- Complete:
  - The digits are fused up to the level of the tips of the fingers.
- Incomplete:
  - Digital fusion does not extend to the tips of the fingers.

- Simple:
  - Only soft-tissue connections are present between the digits.
- Complex:
  - Soft-tissue and bony connections are present between the digits.
- Acrosyndactyly:
  - Complex syndactyly characterized by fusion of the bone distally but not proximally
  - Small spaces (fenestrations) are often present between the digits proximally.

Clinical features

- The middle–ring finger web is the most commonly involved and is affected in approximately 58% of cases.
- The ring–little finger web is affected in 27% of cases.
- The middle–index web is affected in 14% of cases.
- The thumb–index finger web is affected in only 1% of cases.

Indications for surgical correction

- Surgery is not usually performed before 1 year of age.
- Indications for earlier surgery include:
  - Syndactyly between the thumb and index and little and ring fingers.
    - These are generally released earlier as the length discrepancy between these fingers can result in increased deformity with growth.
  - Complex and acrosyndactyly are often released early as the bony connections between digits can adversely affect growth.

Principles of surgical correction

- Many techniques of syndactyly correction have been described.
- Most share the following principles.
  - If multiple digits are involved, the border digits are released first.
  - Single-stage releases of both sides of a digit should be avoided as they may jeopardize finger vascularity.
  - Straight-line incisions along the borders of the digits should be avoided as these have a higher incidence of scar contracture and subsequent digital deformity.
  - The web is generally reconstructed with a proximally based dorsal flap; skin grafts in the web spaces can result in a partial recurrence of syndactyly (web creep).
  - Interdigitating flaps from the volar and dorsal aspects of the digits are used to close the defects along the borders of the digits.
  - There is insufficient skin in all but the most minor cases to directly close all the resultant defects, and full-thickness skin grafts are usually required to resurface these areas.
  - The flaps can be designed so that skin grafts lie solely on one digit.
  - Interdigitating flaps from the hyponychium (the area of finger tip just below the end of the nail) can be used to reconstruct the lateral nail fold.

Camptodactyly

- This condition is characterized by flexion deformity of the proximal interphalangeal joint (PIPJ).
- It most commonly affects the little finger.
- It typically presents during growth spurts which occur:
  - Between 1 and 4 years of age
  - Between 10 and 14 years of age.
- Virtually every structure that passes across the volar aspect of the finger has been implicated in the aetiology of camptodactyly.
- The most common causes are either:
  - An abnormal lumbrical insertion
  - An abnormal flexor digitorum superficialis (FDS) insertion.

Treatment

- Splintage may be helpful in some cases.
- Camptodactyly is a difficult condition to correct surgically and no single procedure has proved to be universally successful.
- It is important to x-ray the finger prior to any surgical intervention.
- Radiological signs that indicate that the deformity may be difficult to correct include:
  - Narrowing of the joint space
  - Indentation of the neck of the proximal phalanx
  - Flattening of the head of the proximal phalanx.
- Some authorities maintain that surgery should be avoided if the condition is mild and the deformity not progressive.
- Surgical options include:
  - Exploration of the digit and release of any tethering structures
    - This may be appropriate in a mild case where the deformity is passively correctable.
  - Angulation osteotomy
  - Arthrodesis (fusion) of the joint.

Trigger thumb

- The clinical signs of trigger thumb in an infant are similar to those seen in an adult.
- 25% of trigger thumbs are present at birth and 25% are bilateral.
- 30% have resolved spontaneously by 1 year of age.
- The child usually holds the thumb in flexion.
- Clicking or triggering is more difficult to elicit in the child than in the adult.
- A nodule (Nottas' node) may be palpable over the tendon of FPL just proximal to the A1 pulley.
- Flexion contractures do occur but correct spontaneously if the triggering resolves or is released before the child is 3 years of age.
- Surgical treatment involves release of the A1 pulley.

Clasped thumb

This is a congenital condition in which the thumb metacarpal is held adducted and the proximal phalanx flexed.

Treatment

- If the extensor tendons are present and the joints supple, splintage in extension for up to 6 months may be successful.
- If there is a significant adduction contracture, relax of the 1st web space release may be indicated.
- Tendon transfers or tendon grafts may be indicated in more severe deformities which remain passively correctable.
- Joint fusions are indicted in severe cases with fixed deformities.

Skeletal failures of differentiation

Clinodactyly

- Clinodactyly is characterized by lateral deformity of the finger.
- It can be differentiated from camptodactyly by the fact that the former contains an 'l' (for lateral) whereas the latter does not.
- Clinodactyly usually affects the little finger and produces radial deviation.
- Clinodactyly may be caused by a triangular-shaped delta phalanx.
- A delta phalanx is formed by an abnormal C-shaped epiphysis, the arm of which extends onto the lateral side of the middle phalanx.
- This abnormal epiphysis is also known as a longitudinal bracketed epiphysis.
- Growth from the longitudinal arm of the epiphysis results in abnormal lateral growth of the bone.

Treatment

- An opening wedge osteotomy is often performed if the finger is short, and closing wedge osteotomy if the finger is long.
- An exchange wedge osteotomy
  - In this procedure, a triangular piece of bone is excised from the longer side of the phalanx and inserted into an opening wedge osteotomy on the short side.

Symphalangism

- Symphalangism was a term used by Harvey Cushing to describe congenital stiffness of the PIPJs.
- Its use has now been extended to include stiffness of the distal interphalangeal joints (DIPJs).
- Symphalangism occurs in association with a number of other conditions including:
  - Apert's syndrome
  - Poland's syndrome
  - Radial club hand.

- Clinical examination reveals absent extension and flexion creases over the affected joints.
- Radiological examination can reveal:
  - Short middle phalanges
  - Poorly developed joints

Treatment

- Symphalangism is usually managed conservatively with physiotherapy and dynamic splintage.
- Arthroplasty or arthrodesis may be considered once skeletal maturity has been attained.

Synostosis

- Synostosis is abnormal fusion of two bones.
- It may be partial, permitting reduced motion, or complete, allowing no motion.
- It can occur at any site in the upper limb where two bones are adjacent to one another.
- Synostosis between the phalanges occurs in complex syndactyly.
- Carpometacarpal, intercarpal and radiocarpal synostosis seldom require any operative intervention.
- Forearm radio-ulnar synostosis is usually functionally handicapping to some extent.
- Rotational osteotomies, placing the hand in a better functional position, can be performed.

Arthrogryposis

- 'Arthrogryposis' is a Greek term meaning 'curved joint'.
- It is thought to be caused by an abnormality in the motor unit of nerves.
- This causes contractures which limit joint mobility during fetal development.
- Clinical findings in patients with arthrogryposis can include:
  - Contractures present at birth and are usually bilateral
  - Adduction and internal rotation of the shoulders
  - Fixed flexion or extension of the elbows and knees
  - Club-like hands and wrists
  - Lack of subcutaneous tissue
  - Thin, waxy skin.
- Treatment begins at a young age and consists of dynamic and static splintage.
- Surgery is sometimes indicated to correct specific functional problems.

Windblown hand

- This is a congenital condition in which the fingers are deviated in an ulnar direction.
- Typically the condition is bilateral and worsens as the child grows.
- Most patients also have an associated 1st web space contracture and a flexion deformity at the metacarpal phalangeal joints.

Treatment

Treatment is usually performed before the child is 2 years of age and involves:

1 Release of the 1st web space contracture

2 Release of the flexor and intrinsic muscles

3 Centralization of the ulnar displaced extensor tendons.

Duplication

- Duplications can involve the whole limb or any part of the limb.
- Polydactyly occurs when more than five fingers are present in a hand.
- Extra digits may be located on the ulnar border, the centre or the radial border of the hand.

Ulnar polydactyly

- Ulnar polydactyly is also known as post-axial polydactyly.
- This is the most common single hand malformation.
- Its incidence is eight times that of polydactyly of the other fingers.
- It is often bilateral.
- Stelling has described the following classification of ulnar polydactyly.
  - *Type 1*: an extra digit attached by a skin bridge only.
  - *Type 2*: an extra digit articulating with the metacarpal or phalanx.
  - *Type 3*: an extra digit articulating with an extra metacarpal.
- Extra digits are usually treated with simple excision.

Central polydactyly

- This usually occurs in conjunction with syndactyly.
- It is frequently bilateral.

Treatment

1 Release of the syndactyly.

2 Excision of the excess tissue.

3 Repair and soft-tissue reconstruction.

Radial polydactyly

- Radial polydactyly is also known as post-axial polydactyly.
- Thumb polydactyly is usually unilateral.
- Typically there is some degree of hypoplasia of both duplicates.
- The radial duplicate is usually the smaller of the two.
- The ulnar-innervated intrinsic muscles to the thumb typically insert onto the ulnar-most thumb duplicate.
- The median-innervated muscles usually insert onto the radial duplicate.
- Wide variations in neurovascular anatomy occur.

Classification

- Wassell has described the following classification of radial polydactyly.
  - *Type 1*: bifid distal phalanx.

- *Type 2*: duplicated distal phalanx.
- *Type 3*: bifid proximal phalanx with duplicated distal phalanx.
- *Type 4*: duplicated proximal and distal phalanx.
- *Type 5*: bifid metacarpal with duplicated proximal and distal phalanx.
- *Type 6*: duplicated metacarpal, proximal and distal phalanx.
- *Type 7*: triphalangeal thumb.

- Type 4 is the commonest abnormality and accounts for approximately 44% of all thumb duplications.

Surgical correction

- Surgical options include:
  1. Removing one duplicate and reconstructing the other.
  2. Removing equal parts of both digits and combining the remaining tissue to form a single finger.
  3. Removing unequal parts of both digits and combining the remaining tissue to form a single finger.
- The first option is used for the most common duplications (Wassell type 4) in which the radial-most digit is proximal and much smaller than its ulnar counterpart.
  - Care must be taken to reconstruct the radial collateral ligaments (RCL).
  - This is usually performed with a periosteal flap taken from the digit to be amputated.
  - The flap is turned down and used to reconstruct the missing RCL.
- The second option is normally used for more distal duplications in which both digits are of similar size.
  - An example is the Bilhaut–Cloquet operation used for Wassell type 1 and 2 deformities.
  - In this operation, the nails are removed and the medial half of each of the duplicate fingers is removed.
  - The remaining outer segments of each digit are then approximated and the nail bed repaired.
  - The original Bilhaut–Cloquet procedure can be modified by taking unequal portions of each finger.
  - In this procedure, the entire nail bed is taken from one of the duplicates.
  - This modification of the Bilhaut–Cloquet operation avoids a central longitudinal nail bed repair and reduces the risk of subsequent nail bed irregularities.

Triphalangeal thumb polydactyly

- In this condition, the thumb has three rather than two phalanges.
- It is relatively common and represents 20% of all thumb polydactylies.
- The extra phalanx may be fully developed or triangular (a delta phalanx).
- Treatment involves removal of the extra phalanx.

Ulnar dimelia

- This rare condition is also known as mirror hand.
- It is characterized by a forearm containing two ulnae but no radial bones.

- The thumb is missing and the hand contains an excessive number of fingers.
- The elbow is usually stiff and forearm rotation reduced.

Treatment
- Excision of the olecranon to increase elbow motility
- Excision of the excess fingers.

Overgrowth

Macrodactyly
- True macrodactyly is characterized by localized enlargement of all structures within a finger.
- This should be distinguished from conditions such as haemangiomas, vascular malformations and Ollier's disease (multiple enchondromatosis) in which only part of the finger is enlarged.
- Macrodactyly is usually unilateral with the index finger being most commonly affected.
- The enlarged area often corresponds to the cutaneous distribution of specific nerves.
- This observation has resulted in the development of an alternative name for this condition—nerve territory orientated macrodactyly.

Classification
Two separate forms of macrodactyly have been described.
1 Static macrodactyly—the enlarged finger grows in proportion to the rest of the child
2 Progressive macrodactyly—the enlarged finger grows out of proportion to the rest of the child.

Surgical correction
- Surgery in areas of macrodactyly is often complicated by delayed healing.
- Surgical options include:
  - Soft-tissue reduction
  - Ablation of the epiphysis (epiphysiodesis)
  - Amputation.

Undergrowth
Hypoplasia of the arm is relatively common and may be associated with Poland's syndrome.

Brachydactyly
Brachydactyly (short fingers) occurs in conditions such as symbrachydactyly in which the fingers are replaced by small nubbins.

Treatment
- Free phalangeal transfers from the toes

- Microvascular free joint or bone transfer
- Distraction.

Thumb hypoplasia

The thumb is the commonest site of clinically significant undergrowth.

Classification

Thumb hypoplasia has been classified by Blauth into five groups.

- *Type 1*
  - A small thumb with normal components
- *Type 2*
  - Hypoplastic thenar muscles
  - Adduction contracture of the first web
  - Laxity of the ulnar collateral ligament (UCL) at the MCPJ
  - Normal skeletal structure.
- *Type 3*
  - Skeletal hypoplasia
  - Hypoplasica of the intrinsic muscles
  - Rudimentary extrinsic tendons
- *Type 4*
  - A small thumb attached to the hand by a soft-tissue bridge
  - This deformity is known as a floating thumb or 'pouce flottant'.
- *Type 5*
  - Total absence of the thumb.

Surgical correction

- Type 1 deformities have good function and do not usually require surgical correction.
- Type 2 deformities are usually treated by release of the 1st web space and an opponensplasty (a muscle transfer to restore thumb opposition).
- The opponensplasty most often used is the Huber transfer in which the distal insertion of the abductor digiti minimi muscle is transferred across the hand to attach to the APB tendon of the thumb.
- Type 3 deformities can either be treated by amputation and pollicization of the index finger or by skeletal and soft-tissue reconstruction.
- Type 4 and 5 deformities are treated by pollicization of the index finger.
- The principles of pollicization are discussed under the treatment of radial club hand (see pp. 197–8).

Constriction ring syndrome

- Constriction rings are tight bands involving all or part of the circumference of hand or digit of the limb.
- The bands are similar to normal skin creases but may extend deeply down to bone.
- The aetiology of constriction bands is not clear but may be due to amniotic bands encircling the limb *in utero*.

Classification
Constriction rings have been subdivided into four groups.
- *Group 1*: a groove in the skin
- *Group 2*: ring constriction with distal lymphoedema
- *Group 3*: ring constriction associated with fusion of distal elements i.e. acrosyndactyly
- *Group 4*: intra-uterine auto-amputation.

Surgical correction
- Excision of the constriction band followed by a soft-tissue release with Z-plasties is used in most cases.
- Traditionally, no more than half of the circumference of the band was released at one time to reduce the risk of distal ischaemia.
- Acrosyndactyly should, if possible, be released in the 1st year of life so that each digit can grow independently.

Nerve compression

- Nerves in the upper limb can be compressed at any point from their site of entry into the arm—the thoracic outlet—to their destination.
- There are certain sites along their courses in which each nerve is particularly prone to compression.
- Factors other than simple compression can produce symptoms; these include:
  - Traction
  - Tethering
  - Excessive excursion
  - Ischaemia.
- Nerve compression typically produces the following symptoms:
  - Pain which can radiate both proximally and distally
  - Sensory disturbance with paraesthesia and numbness
  - Motor disturbance with weakness and wasting.
- On examination the following signs may be present:
  - Tenderness at the site of the nerve compression
  - A positive Tinel's sign at the site of nerve compression
  - Sensory and motor changes distally.

The following are the common sites of nerve compression in the upper limb.

Thoracic outlet syndrome
- This syndrome results from compression of the subclavian vessels and brachial plexus in the base of the neck.
- These structures are typically constricted in the triangle bordered anteriorly by scalenus anterior, posteriorly by scalenus medius and inferiorly by the 1st rib.
- Causes of thoracic outlet syndrome include:
  - Cervical ribs
  - Rudimentary first ribs

- Abnormalities of the scalene muscles
- Bone or soft tissue tumours
- Trauma, i.e. a fractured clavicle
- Poor posture.

· Cervical ribs are present in 0.5% of normal individuals and 10% of patients with thoracic outlet syndrome.

Symptoms

- Symptoms may either be neurogenic or vascular in origin and are often rather vague and ill defined.
- Symptoms may be provoked by certain activities such as carrying heavy loads or working with the arms overhead.
- Neurogenic symptoms predominate and are present in 90% of cases; these include:
  - Pain
  - Paraesthesia
  - Weakness
  - Sympathetic symptoms.
- Vascular symptoms are rarer and occur in approximately 10% of cases; these include:
  - Claudication
  - Splinter haemorrhages and digital emboli
  - Venous engorgement of the limb.

5

Examination

This should include:

1 Assessment of sensation and motor function

2 Auscultation over the subclavian artery with the arms dependent then raised

3 Differential blood pressure measurement between the limbs with the arms dependent then raised

4 Specific provocation tests.

Investigations

These may include:

- Chest and cervical spine x-ray
- CT or MRI scanning to exclude space-occupying lesions
- Angiography or venography.

Management

- Medical
  - Analgesics, carbamazepine, amitriptyline, benzodiazepines and non-steroidal anti-inflammatory drugs (NSAIDs)
  - 75% of patients improve with suitable physiotherapy.
- Surgical
  - Surgical exploration and decompression can be performed via the following approaches.

- Supraclavicular (described by Adson)
- Transaxillary (described by Roos)
- Posterior parascapular (described by Claggett)
- Transthoracic

- Of these, the supraclavicular approach is generally preferred as it provides the best exposure.

The median nerve and its branches

- The median nerve is formed from the continuation of the lateral and medial cords of the brachial plexus.
- It contains fibres from all roots of the brachial plexus (C5-T1).
- It is typically compressed at two sites.
  1. At the elbow—pronator syndrome
  2. Under the flexor retinaculum at the wrist—carpal tunnel syndrome.
- The anterior interosseous branch of the median nerve can be compressed in the forearm.
- This is known as anterior interosseous syndrome.

5

Pronator syndrome

- Pronator syndrome is caused by compression of the median nerve as it travels across the flexor surface of the elbow.
- There are four described anatomical causes of pronator syndrome. From proximal to distal they are:
  1. The ligament of Struthers
     - This arises from a lateral supracondylar process on the lower-third of the humerus.
     - Symptoms are reproduced by resisted elbow flexion.
  2. The lacertus fibrosus
     - This is a fibrous condensation originating from the biceps muscle.
     - Symptoms are reproduced by resisted forearm pronation with the elbow flexed.
  3. The pronator teres
     - Symptoms are reproduced by resisted forearm pronation with the elbow extended.
  4. Under the arch of the FDS
     - Symptoms are reproduced by resisted flexion of the FDS to the middle finger.

Symptoms

Symptoms of pronator syndrome are similar to those of carpal tunnel syndrome with the following exceptions.

- There is altered sensation in the palmar triangle of the palm.
  - This area is supplied by the palmar branch of the median nerve.
  - This nerve arises above the wrist and is therefore unaffected by carpal tunnel syndrome.

- Tinel's sign will not be positive over the carpal tunnel but may be positive over the flexor aspect of the forearm.
- Phalen's test will be negative.
- Nerve-conduction studies will be normal at the wrist.

- Pronator syndrome is treated by decompression.

Carpal tunnel syndrome

- Carpal tunnel syndrome is the most common nerve compression syndrome in the upper limb.
- It occurs in 1–10% of the population.
- Prevalence is reported to be as high as 61% in those who perform repetitive hand movements associated with gripping.

Anatomy

- The base of the carpal tunnel is formed by the bony carpal arch.
- This is bridged by the transverse flexor retinaculum or transverse carpal ligament.
- The flexor retinaculum is attached radially to the tubercle of the scaphoid and the ridge of the trapezium, and ulnarly the hook of the hamate and the pisiform.
- The carpal tunnel contains the nine long flexors to the fingers and thumb and the median nerve.
- At wrist level, the median nerve lies deeply between the FCR and the palmaris longus (PL).

5

Aetiology

- Compression of the median nerve within the carpal tunnel can either be caused by a reduction in the size of the tunnel or an increase in the volume of its contents.
- Reduction in the size of the tunnel can be caused by:
  - Acromegaly
  - Trauma
  - Osteoarthritis (OA).
- Increase in the volume of the contents of the carpal tunnel can be caused by:
  - Swellings, i.e. ganglia or lipomas
  - Inflammation, i.e. tenosynovitis, gout and amyloid
  - Endocrine abnormalities, i.e. pregnancy, diabetes and thyrotoxicosis.
- Congenital causes of carpal tunnel syndrome are rare; these include:
  - A persistent median artery
  - An abnormally long superficial flexor tendon muscle belly
  - An abnormally proximal lumbrical origin
  - The presence of palmaris profundus, an abnormal muscle within the carpal tunnel.

Symptoms

- Symptoms of carpal tunnel syndrome usually include pain, numbness and paraesthesia within the median nerve distribution of the hand.

- Night pain and waking is common and is thought to occur due to the combination of swelling and the flexed position of the wrist adopted in sleep.
- Pain may radiate as far proximally as the shoulder and neck.
- Clumsiness and weakness causing dropping of items is often described.
- Relief of symptoms is often achieved by shaking the hand and placing it in a dependent position.

Clinical features

- There may be wasting and loss of power in the median innervated thenar muscles.
- Altered sensation may be present in the median nerve distribution of the hand.
- Specific provocation tests may be positive.

Provocative tests

- Tinel's sign
  - A positive Tinel's sign is present if percussion over the carpal tunnel induces paraesthesia.
- Phalen's test
  - Phalen's test is positive if flexion of the wrist for 1 min induces paraesthesia.
- The reverse Phalen's test
  - The reverse Phalen's test is positive if extension of the wrist for 1 min induces paraesthesia.
- The carpal compression test
  - The carpal compression test is positive if pressure over the carpal tunnel induces paraesthesia.

Investigations

- Nerve-conduction studies are more sensitive than electromyographic studies.
- Distal latencies are the most sensitive indicators of nerve compression.
- X-ray, CT or MRI is occasionally indicated if there is any suggestion of carpal derangement or space-occupying lesions.

Treatment

- Treatment is either non-operative or operative.
- Non-operative treatments include:
  - Splinting the wrist in a neutral position
  - Steroid injection into the carpal tunnel
  - NSAIDs.
- Surgical decompression of the carpal tunnel can be performed by:
  - An open technique
  - A limited incision technique
  - An endoscopic technique.
- Each technique has its proponents and good results have been reported with each method.
- Some authors recommend that the following procedures be performed in addition to division of the flexor retinaculum.

1 Neurolysis of the median nerve
2 Decompression of the motor branch of the median nerve if there are signs of weakness of the APB
3 Transfer of the PL to the insertion of the APB (Camitz opponensplasty) in patients with thenar wasting.

Anterior interosseous syndrome

- The anterior interosseous nerve branches from the median nerve high in the forearm.
- It is a purely motor nerve and innervates:
  - FPL
  - Flexor digitorum profundus (FDP) to the index and middle fingers
  - Pronator quadratus.
- Symptoms of compression include:
  - Pain
  - Weakness of pinch.
- Signs include:
  - An inability to make an 'O' sign with the thumb and index finger due to paralysis of the long flexors to both the index finger and thumb.
- Sites of compression include:
  - Tendinous bands on either pronator teres (PT) or FDS
  - Gantzer's muscle which is an accessory head of FPL
  - An aberrant radial artery
  - Thrombosis of the ulnar collateral vessel.
- Treatment involves surgical decompression of the offending cause.

5

The ulnar nerve

- The ulnar nerve arises from the medial cord of the brachial plexus.
- It contains fibres from roots C8 and T1.
- The ulnar nerve is typically compressed at one of two sites.
  1 At the elbow—cubital tunnel syndrome
  2 At the wrist in Guyon's canal.

Cubital tunnel syndrome

- The ulnar nerve is compressed as it passes behind the medial epicondyle and into the forearm through Osborne's canal.
- Cubital tunnel syndrome can result from compression of the ulnar nerve by the following:
  - The arcade of Struthers
  - Hypertrophy of the medial head of the triceps
  - The aponeurosis of the flexor carpi ulnaris (FCU)
  - Cubitus valgus (lateral deviation of the elbow)
  - Swellings i.e. lipomata, ganglia or osteophytes
  - Abnormal muscles such as the anconeus epitrochlearis which passes over the nerve from the medial epicondyle to the olecranon.

Symptoms

- Pain which is usually localized to the medial side of the forearm
- Decreased sensation to the ulnar one-and-a-half fingers.

Signs

- Wasting of the hypothenar eminence and clawing of the fingers are rare.
- Tinel's sign may be positive.
- Nerve-conduction studies may be unreliable at this site.

Surgical treatment

- There is some debate over the best method of decompressing the nerve.
- The surgical options include:
  - Simple decompression
  - Anterior transposition of the nerve which can then be placed in either a subcutaneous or submuscular position
  - Medial epicondylectomy.
- Some authorities recommend simple decompression for cases with sensory disturbance only and anterior submuscular transposition for those which have developed motor symptoms.
- During surgery care must be taken to preserve the medial cutaneous nerve of the forearm.

Compression of the ulnar nerve at the wrist

- Guyon's canal is a triangular space superficial to the flexor retinaculum.
- It is traversed by the ulnar artery and nerve.
- Unlike the carpal tunnel, it does not contain any tendons.

Causes

- Repetitive trauma
- Space-occupying lesions such as lipomata, ganglia and aneurysms
- Anomalous muscles such as an accessory PL or an abnormal insertion of the hypothenar muscles
- Fracture of the hook of the hamate.

Symptoms

- Motor loss is the most common sign and results in weakness of the intrinsic muscles.
- Sensory symptoms are less common.

Signs

- Motor signs include:
  - Wasting of the hypothenar eminence
  - An ulnar claw—characterized by hypertension of the MCPs and flexion of the PIPJ and DIPJ
  - Weakness of key pinch
  - A positive Froment's sign.

- Sensory signs include:
  - A positive Tinel's sign
  - Decreased sensation in the ulnar one-and-a-half fingers.

Surgical decompression

- The diagnosis is usually confirmed by nerve-conduction studies prior to surgical intervention.
- Guyon's canal should be decompressed through an incision along the radial border of the FCU.

The radial nerve and its branches

- The radial nerve begins as the continuation of the posterior cord of the brachial plexus.
- It is the largest branch of the brachial plexus.
- It contains fibres from all of the roots of the brachial plexus (C5-T1).
- The radial nerve is typically compressed at the elbow.
- Compression at this site is known as radial tunnel syndrome.
- Its posterior interosseous branch may be compressed in the forearm.
- Its terminal sensory branch—the superficial radial nerve—can be compressed at the wrist.
- This is known as Wartenberg's syndrome.

Radial tunnel syndrome

The radial nerve can be compressed by the following structures at the elbow.

- A fibrous band tethering the nerve to the radiohumeral joint.
- The leash of Henry
  - This consists of radial recurrent vessels which pass across the radial nerve.
- The tendinous margin of extensor carpi radialis brevis (ECRB).
- The arcade of Frohse
  - This is a fibrous band on the surface of the supinator muscle.

Symptoms

- Pain is the predominant symptom and is often confused with that of tennis elbow.
- Motor and sensory disturbance are uncommon.

Signs

- The point of maximum tenderness is typically over supinator four finger breadths distal to the lateral epicondyle.
- The point of maximum tenderness in tennis elbow, in contrast, is located higher over the lateral epicondyle and radial head.
- The middle finger extension test (resisted extension of the middle finger) should be positive in radial tunnel syndrome and negative in tennis elbow.
- Nerve-conduction studies are unreliable and are used to support an essentially clinical diagnosis.

Treatment

Surgical decompression of the radial nerve can be performed through a posterior muscle splitting or anterolateral approach.

Posterior interosseous syndrome

- The posterior interosseous nerve supplies motor innervation to the majority of the forearm extensor musculature.
- It terminates at the wrist as a small sensory branch in the radial side of the base of the 4th extensor compartment.
- The following can cause compression of the nerve.
  - Trauma
    - Dislocation of the elbow
    - Fracture of the radial head
  - Inflammation
    - Rheumatoid arthritis (RA) of the radiohumeral joint
  - Swellings
    - Ganglia and lipomata
  - Iatrogenic
    - After injection for tennis elbow.

5

Symptoms

- The pain is similar in nature to that of radial tunnel syndrome.
- Motor weakness of the forearm extensors is more common than in radial tunnel syndrome.

Signs

- Tenderness may be present over the nerve.
- Tinel's sign may be positive.
- In complete lesions, some wrist extension may be possible as the motor supply to both brachioradialis and extensor carpi radialis longus originates from the radial nerve proximal to its posterior interosseous branch.

Treatment

Posterior interosseous syndrome is treated by surgical decompression.

Compression of the superficial branch of the radial nerve (Wartenberg's syndrome)

- The radial nerve divides into the posterior interosseous and superficial radial nerve approximately 4 cm distal to the lateral epicondyle.
- The superficial radial nerve travels under brachioradialis and becomes superficial in the distal forearm.
- It splits into two or more branches which supply sensation to the dorsum of the thumb, index, middle and radial half of the ring finger.
- The nerve may be compressed at the wrist by bracelets or watches.

Symptoms
Pain in the distribution of the superficial radial nerve which may radiate proximally.

Signs
· Tinel's sign may be positive.
· Percussion over the nerve may produce pain in its cutaneous distribution.

Surgery
· The nerve should be dissected free thoughout its length.
· It may be entrapped by the tendinous margin of brachioradialis, the margin of extensor carpi radialis longus or the fascia between these muscles.

Tendon transfers

General principles

Successful tendon transfer is dependent upon: (i) patient selection; (ii) recipient site factors; (iii) donor site muscle factors; and (iv) surgical technique.

Patient selection

The patient should be:
· Well motivated
· Able to understand the nature and limitations of surgery
· Able to co-operate with post-operative physiotherapy.

Recipient site factors

Ideally the recipient site should have:
· Good soft-tissue coverage without active scar formation
· A stable underlying skeleton
· A full range of passive joint motion
· Normal sensation.

Donor muscle factors

The following factors are important in choosing which muscle to transfer ('APOSLE').

Amplitude of motion
· The donor muscle should have a similar excursion to that which it replaces.
· Excursion of the wrist flexors and extensors is approximately 3 cm.
· Excursion of the finger extensors is approximately 5 cm.
· Excursion of the finger flexors is approximately 7 cm.
· Effective amplitudes of donor tendons can be increased by:
  · Use of the tenodesis effect
  · Freeing fascial attachments to the tendon of the donor muscle unit.

Power and control

- Donor muscles should have a similar pull to those that they replace.
- Muscles with a motor grade of 5 are ideal for transfer.
- Those with a motor grade of 4 function acceptably.
- Transfers of muscles with a motor grade of 3 or less rarely function well.
- Muscles that have been reinervated following injury are not ideal for transfer.
- Some muscles, such as brachioradialis, find it difficult to adapt to their new function.
- As a consequence, the brachioradialis muscle is sometimes called the 'naughty boy' of the wrist.
- Muscles usually lose at least one motor grade following transfer.

One tendon, one function

- Effectiveness of a tendon transfer is reduced when it is expected to produce two different functions.
- Ideally, each tendon transfer should be designed to perform a single action.

Synergistic action

- Muscles which normally act together to produce a composite movement should be used to replace each other whenever possible.
- Finger flexion is usually accompanied by synergistic wrist extension.
- Finger extension is usually accompanied by synergistic wrist flexion.
- A transfer of a wrist flexor to a finger extensor is therefore a synergistic transfer.
- Synergistic transfers function better than asynchronous transfers.

Line of pull

- Tendon transfers function best if they travel directly from their origin to their insertion.
- Deviations from a straight line, such as around a pulley, decrease effectiveness of the transfer.

Expendability

- Only expendable muscles should be transferred.
- For example, it is important that at least one wrist flexor remains intact following tendon transfers to produce wrist and finger extension in patients with radial nerve palsy.

Surgical technique

In general, during tendon transfer surgery, it is important to:

- Operate in reverse order
  - Have the recipient site and tunnel ready before raising the muscle.
- Avoid interference with other structures
  - Care should be taken to ensure that the transferred tendon does not compress other structures, particularly nerves.
- Apply the correct tension

- The ideal tension varies between transfers.
- Extensor indicis (EI) to EPL transfers should be tight as tend to loosen.
- Opponensplasties should be looser to avoid an adduction deformity of the thumb.

Radial nerve palsy

Motor deficits

- Decreased wrist extension
- Decreased finger extension
- Decreased thumb abduction and extension.

Tendon transfers

Classic transfer

- PT to ECRB
- FCU to EDC
- PL to EPL.

Superficialis transfer

- This was described by Boyes as an alternative to the classic transfer.
- It consists of the following:
  - PT to ECRL and ECRB
  - FDS of the middle finger (FDS 3) to EDC
  - FDS of the ring finger (FDS 4) to EIP and EPL
  - FCR to APL and extensor pollicis brevis (EPB).

Median nerve palsy

Motor deficits

- The main functional deficit is lack of thumb opposition due to denervation of the thenar eminence.
- APB is the thenar eminence muscle most reliably supplied by the median nerve.
- Flexor pollicis brevis (FPB) and opponens pollicis are often partially supplied by the ulnar nerve.
- Consequently, some patients with low median nerve palsies still have adequate thumb opposition.

Tendon transfers

Tendon transfers to restore thumb opposition are known as opponensplasties. There are four main types of opponensplasty.

The Royle–Thompson opponensplasty

- FDS 4 is divided at its distal attachment.

- The tendon is then passed superficially through the palmar fascia at which point it pivots before crossing the palm.
- The tendon is then attached onto the insertions of APB or EPB.

The extensor indices transfer

The EI is re-routed around the ulnar side of the hand and inserted into the insertion of APB or EPB.

The Camitz transfer

- PL is lengthened with a strip of palmar fascia and attached to the insertion of APB.
- This transfer is particularly useful in long-standing median nerve palsy and is often combined with carpal tunnel release in older patients.

The Huber transfer

- The abductor digiti minimi is detached distally and elevated preserving its proximal neurovascular supply.
- The muscle is then transposed across the palm and inserted into the insertion of APB or EPB.

Ulnar nerve palsy

Motor deficits

Ulnar nerve palsy is characterized by weakness of:

- Thumb adduction due to paralysis of the adductor pollicis.
- Paralysis of the **d**orsal interossei causing weakness in finger **ab**duction ('DAB').
- Paralysis of the **p**almar interossei causing weakness in finger **add**uction ('PADD').
- Ulnar clawing
  - Clawing is the combination of hyperextension of the MCPJs and flexion of the interphalangeal joints (IPJs).
  - This is caused by weakness of intrinsic muscles (interossei and lumbricals) which pulls on the extensor mechanism straightening the IPJs.
  - Hyperextension of the MCPJs occurs due to pull of the EDC tendons.
  - The EDC muscle is unaffected by ulnar nerve palsy as it is innervated by the posterior interosseous nerve.
  - Low ulnar palsy results in a more pronounced claw than higher lesions (this is known as the ulnar paradox).
  - Low lesions cause a greater claw because the ulnarly innervated long flexors to the ring and little fingers produce PIP and DIP flexion.
  - In high lesions, these muscles are denervated and therefore do not increase finger flexion at the IPJs.

Tendon transfers

Loss of thumb adduction

- FDS 3 or 4 can be detached distally and attached to the insertion of the adductor pollicis.

· ECRB can be lengthened with a tendon graft and inserted onto the adductor tubercle of the thumb.
· Brachioradialis can be extended with a tendon graft and passed into the palm from the dorsum through the 3rd web space. It is then attached to the insertion of the adductor pollicis.

Claw deformity
· Any surgical procedure which limits MCPJ hyperextension will control the claw deformity.
· Many techniques have been described.
· Zancolli's lasso technique is one of the most commonly used.
· In this technique, FDS slips are divided at their insertion, reflected proximally, volar to the A1 pulley, and attached proximally to themselves.
· This 'lasso' around the A1 pulley limits extension of the MCPJs.

Dupuytren's disease

Dupuytren's disease is a condition of unknown aetiology characterized by contraction of the palmar or digital fascia.

Incidence
· Dupuytren's disease affects 1–3% of the population of North Europe and the USA.
· It is rare in the Far East and Africa.
· It is three times as common in males.
· Its incidence increases with age.
· It has a strong hereditary disposition.

Aetiology
· The cause of Dupuytren's disease is unknown.
· It is more common in patients with diabetes, liver disease, epilepsy and TB.
· It may be associated with a high alcohol intake and local trauma.
· Workers known to be at risk are:
  · Jockeys
  · Trombone players
  · Pneumatic drill operators.
· There appears to be different patterns of disease.
  · Diabetics and people of Oriental extraction tend to develop palmar disease.
  · Patients with Dupuytren's diathesis often have a strong family history and bilateral aggressive disease which is prone to recurrence.

Pathogenesis
· In the early stages of the disease a large number of fibroblasts are present in the palmar fascia.
· They are believed to transform into myofibroblasts.

- Myofibroblasts contain smooth muscle fibres and may be responsible for the contraction noted in Dupuytren's disease.
- Type 3 collagen predominates in the early phases of the disease.
- The proportion of type 1 collagen increases as the condition progresses.

Associated conditions

Conditions associated with Dupuytren's disease include:
- Knuckle pads—Garrod's pads
- Penile fibrous plaques—Peyronie's disease
- Plantar fibromatosis—Lederhosen's disease.

Anatomy of the palmar and digital fascia

- Normal fascial structures are referred to as fascial bands.
- Diseased fascial structures are referred to as cords.
- The palmar aponeurosis is made up of three layers.
  1 A superficial layer containing longitudinal fibres
  2 An intermediate layer containing transverse fibres
  3 A deep layer containing vertical fibres binding it to the metacarpals.
- Distally the longitudinal fibres split into three layers and insert:
  1 Superficially into the skin of the palm
  2 Into the spiral band of Gosset which passes into the lateral digital sheet
  3 Deeply into the middle phalanx and flexor sheath.
- The spiral band is a normal condensation of fascia that extends from the longitudinal fibres of the palmar fascia to the natatory ligament.
- The natatory ligament passes transversely across the web space; its contracture limits separation of the fingers.
- The lateral digital sheets are condensations of fascia that run vertically along the finger outside the neurovascular bundle.
- Grayson's ligaments pass laterally from the proximal and middle phalanx to the skin volar to the neurovascular bundles.
- Cleland's ligaments pass laterally from the proximal and middle phalanx to the skin dorsal to the neurovascular bundles.
- Cleland's ligaments are said never to be involved in Dupuytren's disease.
- *Aide-mémoire*—Cleland's ligaments are **d**orsal.

Anatomy of the diseased palmar and digital fascia

- A pretendinous cord is a contracture of the superficial longitudinal layer of the palmar fascia.
- A central cord is a continuation of the pretendinous cord into the finger.
- A lateral cord is a contracture of the lateral digital sheets.
- An abductor digiti minimi cord is often present on the ulnar side of the little finger.
- A spiral cord is made up of the following four elements from proximal to distal.
  1 A pretendinous cord
  2 A spiral cord

3 The lateral digital sheet
4 Grayson's ligament.
- It forms a tight cord attached proximally to the palmar fascia and distally to the middle phalanx.
- Spiral cords are in fact straight.
- As they contract they cause the neurovascular bundles to spiral medially and superficially.
- A more correct term might be spiral nerve and artery.
- The presence of a spiral cord increases the risk of iatrogenic damage during surgery.
- Care must be taken at the level of the MCP to identify displaced nerves and vessels.

Indications for surgical treatment

- Indications for surgical intervention in Dupuytren's disease include:
  - Flexion deformity of the MCPJs of more than 20–30°
  - Any contracture of the IPJs
  - Painful nodules
  - Rapidly progressive disease
  - A strong family history of aggressive disease.
- Moderate flexion of the MCPJs is not an indication for surgery as the collateral ligaments of the MCPJs are stretched in a flexed position.
- In contrast, the collateral ligaments of the IPJs are relaxed in a flexed position.
- This allows them to shorten resulting in a fixed flexion deformity.
- Flexion of the IPJs is therefore a stronger indication for surgery than flexion of the MCPJs.

Surgical approaches

Surgical techniques for treating Dupuytren's disease vary in: (i) the pattern of skin incision or excision; and (ii) the amount of fascia resected.

Skin incision/excision

Longitudinal incision

A number of incisions have been described to access the diseased fascia, including:
- A straight-line incision broken up with Z-plasties, as described by Skoog
- A zigzag incision, as described by Brunner
- An incision incorporating multiple V-Y plasties, as described by Palmen.

Transverse incision

- Transverse incisions are generally used if the diseased fascia affects more than one ray.
- A transverse incision with extension into the fingers was described by Skoog.
- The open palm technique in which the transverse palm wound was left to heal by secondary intention was described by McCash.

Skin excision
· Excision of adherent skin with the underlying diseased fascia (dermofasciectomy) is advocated by some for rapidly progressive or recurrent disease.
· The resultant defect is usually reconstructed with a full-thickness skin graft.

Fascia resection

Fasciotomy
· Simple division of the diseased cords may be indicated in patients unsuitable for more radical procedures.
· This can be performed without a skin incision using the sharp end of a needle.

Fasciectomy
· Elective regional fasciectomy involves excision of the diseased fascia.
· The transverse fibres of the palmar fascia are retained.
· A limited regional fasciectomy involves removal of all of the palmar fascia leading to a single digit.
· A radical fasciectomy involves removal of all the palmar fascia.

Releasing fixed flexion deformities of the PIPJ
· Even after all the diseased fascia has been removed, a fixed flexion deformity of the PIPJ may remain.
· The following manoeuvres may be used to release the flexion deformity.

1. Transverse incision of the flexor sheath
2. Release of the check rein ligaments (fibrous condensations between the volar plate and the proximal phalanx).
3. Collateral ligament release
4. Volar capsulotomy.

Post-operative management
Important factors in the post-operative management include:
· Elevation
· Splintage immediately after surgery
· Physiotherapy
· Dynamic splinting in some cases
· The use of a static resting night splint for up to 6 months following surgery.

Tumours
Tumours of the hand can arise from any of its constituent tissues.

Skin
· Benign non-pigmented lesions
· Benign pigmented lesions
· Malignant non-pigmented lesions
· Malignant pigmented lesions.

Fat
- Lipoma
- Angiolipoma
- Liposarcoma.

Vascular tissue
- Haemangiomas
- Vascular malformations
- Glomus tumours
- Aneurysms
- Angio- or lymphangiosarcoma
- Kaposi's sarcoma.

Muscle
- Leiomyoma
- Leiomyosarcoma
- Rhabdomyosarcoma.

Fibrous tissue
- Dupuytren's nodules
- Dermatofibroma
- Dermatofibrosarcoma protuberans
- Fibroxanthoma
- Fibrosarcoma.

Neural tissue
- Neuroma
- Glioma
- Neurofibroma
- Neurilemmoma
- Neurosarcoma
- Merkel cell tumour.

Tendon sheath
- Rheumatoid synovitis
- Trigger finger nodules
- Giant cell tumours of the tendon sheath
- Joint
- Ganglia.

Bone and cartilage
- Enchondroma
- Osteochondroma
- Osteoid osteoma
- Simple bone cysts

- Aneurysmal bone cyst
- Giant cell tumour of bone
- Chondrosarcoma
- Osteogenic sarcoma
- Ewing's sarcoma
- Metastatic tumour.

Many of these conditions are not unique to the hand. Of the above, the following tumours are most common.

Ganglia

- Ganglia are the commonest soft-tissue tumour of the hand and account for 50–70% of all lesions.
- Ganglia are three times as common in women.
- 70% of ganglia present between 20 and 40 years of age.

Pathogenesis

- There is some debate as to the cause of ganglia.
- Possible causes include:
  - Herniation of the joint capsule, as described by Volkmann in 1872
  - Ligament strain resulting in mucinous degeneration
  - Embryological remnants of synovial tissue in the joint capsule.

Location

- The four most common types of ganglion are:
  1. Dorsal wrist ganglia
  2. Volar wrist ganglia
  3. Ganglia of the flexor sheath (volar retinacular ganglia)
  4. Mucous cysts (ganglia of the DIPJ).
- Ganglia can also occur in the following sites.
  - Over the PIPJ
  - Over the extensor tendon
  - Within Guyon's canal
  - Within the carpal tunnel
  - Within bone (interosseous ganglion).

Signs and symptoms

- Many ganglia are asymptomatic.
- Presenting symptoms may include:
  - A dull ache
  - Weakness of the hand or wrist (due to carpal involvement or nerve compression).

Differential diagnosis

The following conditions can be confused with a ganglion.

Carpometacarpal boss

- This is an osteoarthritic spur which develops over the CMCJ of the index or middle fingers.
- It presents as a hard, immobile and occasionally tender lump.
- A carpometacarpal boss frequently occurs in conjunction with a dorsal wrist ganglion.

Extensor digitorum manus brevis

- This is an abnormal accessory muscle.
- Aching pain in a similar distribution to that of a dorsal wrist ganglion may occur.

Dorsal wrist ganglia

- These account for 60–70% of all hand ganglia.
- They originate from the scapholunate ligament (SLL).
- They may present anywhere on the back of the hand.
- Dissection reveals a connection with the SLL via a pedicle.
- This pedicle typically emerges from between the EPL and the EDC.
- Occult SLL ganglia are small and are often difficult to detect clinically.
- They may cause wrist pain by exerting pressure on the SLL.
- Diagnosis of occult SLL ganglia is usually made by ultrasound.

Treatment

Dorsal wrist ganglia can be managed: (i) non-surgically; and (ii) surgically.

Non-surgical management

- Benign neglect—approximately 40% will resolve spontaneously
- Sclerosant therapy
- Aspiration
- Intralesional steroid injections
- Pressure.

Surgical excision

- A transverse incision is made over the SLL.
- The EPL and EDC tendons are then retracted radially and ulnarly, respectively, and the pedicle is mobilized down to the underlying joint capsule.
- The capsule is then incised and the ganglion is tangentially excised off the SLL.
- Recurrence rates of up to 40% have been reported after surgical excision.

Volar wrist ganglia

- These account for approximately 20% of all hand ganglia.
- Volar wrist ganglia typically originate from the scaphotrapezium-trapezoid (STT) joint.

5

- Volar wrist ganglia usually pass superficially radial to the FCR.
- Most volar wrist ganglia are closely related and may be attached to the radial artery.

Treatment
- Surgical excision is usually recommended.
- Aspiration and injection may result in damage to the radial artery.
- It is important to perform an Allen's test prior to surgery to test the adequacy of the ulnar arterial supply to the hand.
- Longitudinal or transverse incisions may be used.
- The pedicle of the ganglion is dissected with care to protect the radial artery.
- The ganglion is then tangentially excised at its origin.

Ganglia of the flexor sheath
- Ganglia of the flexor sheath are also known as volar retinacular ganglia.
- They account for approximately 10% of hand ganglia.
- Flexor sheath ganglia present as firm, immobile tender masses at the level of the proximal digital crease.
- They arise from the A1 pulley and do not move with the tendon.
- They occur most frequently in the middle finger.

Treatment
- Attempts at needle rupture followed by steroid injection are recommended prior to surgery.
- A variety of incisions have been described.
- The neurovascular bundles should be identified and preserved.
- The ganglion should be excised with a small portion of underlying A1 pulley.

Mucous cysts
- Mucous cysts arise from the DIPJ.
- They usually occur between the 5th and 7th decades.
- The earliest clinical sign is often longitudinal nail grooving due to pressure on the germinal matrix.
- Later a swelling may appear between the distal joint crease and the base of the nail.
- The patient may also have Heberden's nodes and radiological evidence of OA in the DIPJ.

Treatment
- An L-shaped or curved incision is made over the cyst.
- The cyst is then mobilized and traced proximally where it is excised with a portion of joint capsule.
- Care is taken to preserve the extensor insertion proximally and the germinal matrix of the nail distally.
- A local flap or skin graft may be required if a significant amount of skin is excised.

Giant cell tumours of the tendon sheath

- This lesion is also known as localized pigmented villonodular tenovagosynovitis.
- It is a relatively common, soft-tissue tumour of the hand.
- Although it is a benign tumour it can be locally invasive.
- It typically presents as a painless mass on the palmar surface of the fingers, hand or wrist.
- The tumour is typically grey and multiloculated.
- Treatment is by local excision.
- Complete local excision is often difficult and recurrence is common.

Glomus tumours

- A glomus is an arteriovenous anastomosis involved in thermoregulation.
- A large number are present beneath the nails and in finger pulps.
- Patients with glomus tumours typically present with the triad of:
  1. Pain
  2. Tenderness
  3. Cold insensitivity.
- Clinically, glomus tumours resemble a small haemangioma.
- If located on the nail bed, ridging of the nail may be present.
- The following clinical signs may be present.
  - Love's sign is the presence of one exquisitely painful spot on palpation.
  - Hildred's sign is a reduction of pain on exsanguination of the affected part.
- Treatment is by surgical excision.

Bone and cartilage tumours

Enchondroma

- An enchondroma is an area of abnormal cartilage formation within a bone.
- These slow-growing, benign lesions are the most common primary tumours of the hand.
- They are usually located in either the phalanges or metacarpals.
- They often present as pathological fractures following minimal trauma in young adults.
- The lesions classically have the following radiological appearance.
  - A central radiolucent area
  - Thinning and expansion of the bony cortex
  - Speckled calcification within the radiolucent area.
- Treatment is curettage and bone grafting.
- Multiple enchondromatosis is known as Ollier's disease.
- In this condition the enchondromas tend to be larger and are often associated with skeletal deformity.
- They can differentiate into chondrosarcomas and any sudden change in their behaviour warrants biopsy.
- Maffucci's syndrome consists of multiple enchondromas associated with vascular anomalies.

Osteochondroma

- These are benign bony tumours commonly found in the radius and ulna.
- The lesions are known as osteochondromas if they are capped by cartilage.
- The risk of malignant transformation is very low.
- Functional impairment is common and is the main indication for surgery.

Osteoid osteoma

- These are a benign bone-forming tumours which usually occur in the young.
- They are characterized by pain relieved by aspirin.
- Diagnosis is often difficult as the radiological changes are often subtle.
- The characteristic appearances on x-ray are:
  - A lesion <1 cm in diameter
  - A small central sclerotic nidus surrounded by a lucent zone
  - A sclerotic rim.
- Treatment is by curettage with or without bone grafting.

Simple bone cysts

- These are benign cystic lesions.
- They are commonly located in the distal radius.
- Treatment options include:
  - Aspiration and steroid injection
  - Curettage.

Aneurysmal bone cyst

- These rare tumours tend to occur in the 2nd and 3rd decades.
- Although benign, they may invade locally and are prone to local recurrence following excision.
- *En bloc* resection is recommended to minimize the risk of recurrence.

Arthritis

- Rheumatic disorders include all painful conditions of the locomotor system.
- Rheumatism is a lay term for any pain related to the musculoskeletal system.
- Arthritis is joint disease associated with inflammation.

Arthritic diseases of the upper extremity can be subdivided into the following main groups.

Degenerative arthritis

Erosive arthritis (osteoarthritis).

Inflammatory arthritis

- RA
- Psoriatic arthritis
- Gout

- Pseudogout
- Systemic lupus erythematosus (SLE).

Infective arthritis
Septic arthritis.

Osteoarthritis

Incidence

- 10% of adults over 50 years of age have some degree of OA.
- Radiological evidence of OA is present in almost everyone over 60 years of age.

Pathogenesis

- OA is characterized by destruction of articular cartilage.
- Most of the periarticular bone surrounding joints with OA is sclerotic, however, it may contain areas of relative porosity (cysts).
- Mild synovitis and inflammatory joint effusions are often present.
- Most cases are idiopathic but the following factors predispose the premature development of OA.
  - Joint injury
  - Joint instability
  - Joint surgery
  - Inflammatory joint disease.

Clinical features

- The joints of the upper limb most commonly affected by OA are:
  - The DIPJs
  - The basal joints of the thumb.
- Pain stiffness and limitation of movement are the most common symptoms.
- Joint examination reveals bony swelling (due to osteophytes), effusions and tenderness.
- Bony swellings at the DIPJs are known as Heberden's nodes while those at the PIPJ are referred to as Bouchard's nodes.

Radiological features

Classical radiological features of joints affected by OA include:

- Narrowing of the joint space
- Sclerosis and cyst formation within the bone underlying the joint
- Periarticular osteophyte formation.

Treatment

Non-operative

- Splintage
- NSAIDs

- Intra-articular steroid injections
- Physiotherapy.

Operative

- While operative options for the DIPJ are relatively limited multitiple operations have been described for OA of the CMCJ.
- Surgical options for the CMCJ include:
  - Arthrodesis
  - Osteotomy of the base of the first metacarpal
  - Trapeziumectomy
  - Ligament reconstruction.
- Of these, trapeziumectomy is probably the most commonly performed.
- The defect produced on removing the trapezium can be filled with:
  - An implant
  - A segment of rolled-up FCR
  - A segment of palmaris longus.

Rheumatoid arthritis

RA is characterized by inflammation and proliferation of synovium.

Incidence

- RA affects 2% of the population worldwide.
- It is three times as common in females.
- 90% of patients have some degree of hand involvement.
- 10% have significant hand involvement.

Aetiology

- The precise cause of RA is unknown.
- It is thought to be due to an autoimmune reaction to an unknown agent within the synovial tissue.
- This antigen interacts with IgG and IgM antibodies to produce synovial inflammation.
- 70% of patients are rheumatoid factor positive, i.e. they have IgG or IgM auto-antibodies in their serum.

Classification

- RA can be classified anatomically by the number of joints affected.
  - Monoarthropathy—one joint affected
  - Pauciarthropathy—two to four joints affected
  - Polyarthropathy—over four joints affected.
- It may be classified by its clinical course into:
  - Monocyclic disease—one attack
  - Polycyclic disease—recurrent attacks
  - Progressive disease—chronic worsening disease.
- The condition is characterized by three distinct phases.

1 Proliferation—synovial swelling and pain
2 Destruction—erosion of tendon, bone and joint
3 Reparation—decreased synovial activity and fibrosis.

Non-articular manifestations

RA can be considered a multiple organ disease as it can also involve the following systems.

The eyes

- Iritis, scleritis and uveitis can occur.
- Sjögren's syndrome is the triad of:
  1 Dry eyes (keratoconjunctivitis sicca)
  2 Dry mouth (xerostomia)
  3 RA.

The nervous system

- Polyneuropathy
- Carpal tunnel syndrome.

The haemopoetic system

- Anaemia is commonly associated with RA.
- Felty's syndrome is RA associated with splenomegaly and neutropenia.

The heart

Pericarditis, myocarditis and pericardial effusions may be present.

The lungs

- Pleural effusions
- Rheumatoid nodules can occur within the lungs.
- Caplan's syndrome consists of nodular pulmonary fibrosis in patients with RA exposed to industrial dusts.

The kidneys

RA is a common cause of amyloidosis affecting the kidneys.

The skin

- Vasculitic ulcers
- Pretibial lacerations due to thinning of skin secondary to steroid administration
- Rheumatoid nodules are present in approximately 20% of patients with RA.
- These soft-tissue swellings can occur anywhere but are particularly common over the ulnar just distal to the elbow.

Clinical presentation

- Patients may present with joint or systemic symptoms.
- The following upper-limb joints are frequently affected.

- The elbow
- The wrist
- The MCPJs
- The PIPJs.
- It is important to record:
  - The time period over which the symptoms have occurred
  - The degree of functional impairment.

Investigation

- Blood should be tested for rheumatoid factors.
- Classical radiological appearances of RA include:
  - Narrowing of the joint space
  - Erosions on the surface of the joint
  - Soft-tissue swelling
  - Cysts within the periarticular bone
  - Generalized osteoporosis.

Non-operative treatment

- First-line drug treatment includes:
  - NSAIDs
  - Corticosteroids
- Second-line drug treatment includes:
  - Azathioprine
  - Gold compounds
  - Hydrochloroquinone.
- Steroid injections, physiotherapy and splintage may also be useful.

Operative treatment

- Indications for surgery, in order of importance, are:
  1. Relief of pain
  2. Improvement of function
  3. Prophylactic surgery to prevent future deformity
  4. Surgery to improve the cosmetic deformity.
- Deformity without functional loss is not an indication for surgery.
- Surgical options for most deformities include:
  - Synovectomy
  - Arthroplasty
  - Arthrodesis
  - Tendon repair, replacement or repositioning.

The wrist

- The classic wrist deformity is caput ulnae syndrome.
- This consists of:
  - Volar subluxation of the carpus from the ulnar
  - Volar subluxation of the extensor carpi ulnaris (ECU)
  - Supination of the carpus.

- Findings on examination include:
  - A prominent ulnar which depresses and then lifts on pressure (the piano key sign)
  - Dorsal swelling due to synovial proliferation within the extensor compartments.
- Surgical options include:
  - Distal ulnar excision (Darrach procedure)
  - Transfer of the tendons of ECRL or ECU
  - Wrist fusion.

Dorsal tenosynovitis

- Proliferative synovitis within the extensor compartment at the wrist presents as a boggy swelling which extends proximally and distally.
- Extensor tendon rupture may occur due to:
  - Synovial infiltration of the tendons.
  - Abrasion of the EDC on the ulnar styloid and distal radio-ulnar joint (DRUJ) (Vaughan–Jackson lesion).
  - Abrasion of EPL on Lister's tubercle.
- Dorsal synovectomy is indicated in cases with significant swelling unresponsive to medical treatment.
- After completion of the synovectomy, the extensor retinaculum is placed under, rather than over, the tendons.
- This has the following advantages.
  - It provides a smooth surface on which the tendons can glide.
  - It protects the tendons from future synovial infiltration.

Extensor tendon rupture

- Extensor tendon rupture tends to occur in an ulnar-to-radial direction commencing in the little finger.
- Direct repair is usually impossible as the tendon edges are usually rather frayed.
- Suture of the distal portion to the intact neighbouring ring finger extensor is the operation of choice.
- Ruptures of both little and ring finger extensors can be repaired by:
  - Suturing the distal ends of both to the intact middle finger extensor.
  - Suturing the distal end of the ring finger tendon to the intact middle finger extensor and reconstructing the little finger extensor with an EI transfer.
- If more tendons are ruptured, cross-linking with the remaining intact extensors is performed.
- If all the tendons are ruptured, FDS-4 can be transferred from the palm and sutured to the distal extensors (Boyes transfer).

Flexor tenosynovitis

- Typically, flexor tenosynovitis presents with:
  - Pain on finger flexion
  - Decreased range of finger movement.
- Trigger finger and carpal tunnel may occur.
- Clinically, crepitus can be felt on finger flexion.
- Synovial erosion may result in flexor tendon rupture.

- At surgery, small nodules (rice bodies) may be found within the flexor sheaths.
- Treatment is by flexor synovectomy.

Flexor tendon rupture
- The FPL tendon is the most commonly ruptured flexor tendon.
- This usually occurs due to attrition from osteophytes on the scaphoid (Mannerfelt lesion).
- Reconstruction is performed by one of the following techniques.
  - Direct repair
  - Tendon graft
  - FDS transfer.
- Rupture of other flexor tendons are treated in the following ways.
  - FDP rupture in the palm
    - Transfer of the distal tendon stump to the adjacent FDP
  - FDP rupture in the finger
    - Stabilization of the DIPJ combined with tenosynovectomy to preserve FDS function
  - FDS
    - This rupture is not always recognized as there is little functional impairment
    - Synovectomy may be performed to protect the FDP.

Metacarpophalangeal joints
- In rheumatoid disease the MPJs sublux in a volar and ulnar direction.
- Factors responsible for volar subluxation include:
  - A weak or stretched dorsal extensor expansion
  - Dislocation of the extensor tendons into the valleys between the metacarpals
  - Detached or stretched collateral ligaments.
- Factors responsible for ulnar deviation of the fingers include:
  - Thumb pressure on the index finger from key pinch
  - Intrinsic tendon tightness
  - The pull of abductor digiti minimi
  - Ulnar inclination of the heads of the metacarpals.
  - Radial deviation of the wrist
  - Ulnar deviating forces of the flexor tendons
- Surgical options for MCPJ disease include:
  - Synovectomy
  - Synovectomy combined with soft-tissue reconstruction including:
    - Intrinsic release
    - Crossed intrinsic transfer
    - Extensor tendon stabilization
  - Replacement arthoplasty.

Proximal interphalangeal joints
- Synovial inflammation and proliferation results in stretching of the extensor mechanism.

- The resultant imbalance in the extensor mechanism produces either a swan neck or boutonnière deformity.

Swan neck deformity

- This is characterized by hyperextension at the PIPJ and flexion at the DIPJ.
- The exact cause of the deformity is unclear but contributory factors include:
  - Volar plate rupture
  - Attenuation of FDS
  - Intrinsic tightness.
- Surgical treatment depends on the mobility of the PIPJ.
  - PIPJ flexible in all positions—splint-limiting extension or FDS sling
  - PIPJ flexion limited—intrinsic release, extensor tenolysis, capsulodesis or tenodesis
  - Stiff PIPJ with joint destruction—arthroplasty or arthrodesis.

Boutonnière deformity

- The boutonnière deformity is so called because it is said to resemble an old-fashioned device for doing up buttons.
- The deformity is characterized by flexion at the PIPJ and extension at the DIPJ.
- Synovial proliferation erodes the weakest part of the extensor mechanism just lateral to the central slips over the PIPJ.
- This results in lateral displacement of the lateral bands which then exert a flexor rather than an extensor force on the PIPJ.
- Surgical correction is difficult and is associated with a high-recurrence rate.
- The following operations have been described.
  - Early deformity
    - Synovectomy
    - Reattachment of the central slip
    - Relocation of the lateral bands
  - Late deformity
    - Arthrodesis or athroplasty.

The thumb

- Nalebuff has classified thumb deformities into four groups.
  - *Group 1*: flexion at the MCPJ (boutonnière deformity)
  - *Group 2*: flexion at the MCPJ with the metacarpal adducted
  - *Group 3*: zigzag deformity (a Z-shaped thumb)
    - The CMCJs and IPJs are flexed.
    - The MCP joint is extended.
    - Similar to a swan neck deformity
  - *Group 4*: gamekeeper's thumb
    - The CMCJ is subluxed.
    - The ulnar collateral ligament of the MCPJ is attenuated or ruptured.
- Treatment is aimed towards correcting the underlying abnormality.

- As in most rheumatoid conditions, surgery consists of one, or a combination, of the following.
  - Synovectomy
  - Arthroplasty
  - Arthrodesis
  - Tendon repair, replacement or repositioning.

Psoriatic arthropathy

- Approximately 10% of patients with this common skin disease develop inflammatory arthritis.
- Clinically, this is characterized by:
  - Involvement of the DIPJs
  - Acute attacks affecting the entire finger and toe (sausage finger).
- Radiological features include:
  - Joint surface erosions
  - A concave cup deformity of the articular surface of the distal phalanx
  - A convex pencil deformity of the articular surface of the middle phalanx at the DIPJ.

Gout

- Males are affected eight times more commonly than females.
- Gout is caused by intra- and periarticular deposition of needle-shaped crystals of monosodium urate monohydrate (MUM).
- Intra- and periarticular deposition of MUM crystals initiates an inflammatory arthritis.
- Pseudo-gout is caused by intra-articular deposits of calcium pyrophosphate.
- MUM is derived from uric acid.
- Hyperuricaemia may be primary or secondary.
- Causes of primary hyperuricaemia include:
  - Increased dietary intake (classically red wine and meat)
  - Enzyme abnormalities
  - Decreased secretion by the gut and kidneys.
- Causes of secondary hyperuricaemia include:
  - Diuretics (particularly thiazides)
  - Myeloproliferative disorders.

Clinical presentation

Acute gout

- Acute attacks of gout cause painful synovitis.
- 90% of attacks are self limiting.
- 60% affect the first metatarsophalangeal joint.
- The wrists and fingers are often involved.
- Affected areas become red and inflamed.
- Clinically, the main differential diagnosis is infection.

Chronic tophaceous gout

- Patients develop subcutaneous nodules containing crystals.
- These may ulcerate through the skin.
- Tophaceous gout may be accompanied by erosive arthritis.

Diagnosis

- This is based on the identification of MUM crystals by polarized light microscopy.
- High uric acid levels are not diagnostic of gout.
- Most patients with gout have hyperuricaemia, however, most patients with hyperuricaemia do not have gout.
- Typical radiological appearances include:
  - Large punched-out erosions away from the joint margin
  - Soft-tissue swelling.

Treatment

- Acute gout is treated by:
  - High-dose NSAIDs
  - Colchicine
- Chronic gout is treated by:
  - Low-purine diets
  - The xanthine oxidase inhibitor allopurinol
  - Uricosuric drugs such as probenecid.

Hand infections

Microbiology

- The most common pathogen in hand infections is *Staphylococcus aureus.*
- Bite wounds contaminated with human saliva contain a mixture of aerobic and anaerobic bacteria.
- Aerobic pathogens include:
  - *Staphylococcus aureus*
  - *Staphylococcus epidermidis*
  - *Streptococci.*
- Anaerobic pathogens include:
  - *Peptostreptococci*
  - *Peptococci*
  - *Bacteroides*
  - *Eikenella corrodens.*
- Cat and dog bites are frequently colonized by *Pasteurella multocida.*

Acute paronychia

- Paronychia is infection of the soft tissue just proximal to the nail fold.
- It is the most common hand infection.
- The first clinical signs of infection are pain and erythema.
- Later, a collection may form between the germinal matrix and the overlying skin.
- This collection should be drained by either:
  - Gently separating the nail from the eponychial fold; or
  - An incision over the collection.

Chronic paronychia

- This chronic inflammatory condition results in thickening of the cuticle and grooving of the nail.
- It is most commonly seen in middle-aged women.
- The causative organism in many of these cases is *Candida albicans.*
- Effective treatment is difficult and may consist of:
  - Marsupialization of the eponychium
  - Nail removal followed by application of antifungal cream to the nail bed.

Felon

- This is an infection of the finger pulp.
- It usually occurs as a result of a penetrating wound.
- The resultant abscess results in pain and erythema.
- The collection should be drained over the point of maximum fluctuance.
- Untreated infections may result in:
  - Osteomyelitis
  - Septic arthritis
  - Flexor sheath infections
  - Tender scars on the finger pulp.

Herpetic whitlow

- This is a superficial infection of the finger tip.
- It is caused by the herpes simplex virus.
- It is common in health workers, such as dentists, who are exposed to the virus.
- It typically presents with pain, swelling and erythema of the affected finger.
- Small clear vesicles are present at the early stages of the infection.
- Treatment is conservative and the infection typically resolves within 3 weeks.
- Surgical drainage is **not** indicated as this can result in a bacterial superinfection.

Flexor sheath infections

- These severe infections usually occur as a result of a penetrating injury to the flexor sheath.
- Kanavel described the four cardinal signs of flexor sheath infection.
  1. Fusiform swelling of the finger
  2. Semi-flexed finger position
  3. Tenderness over the flexor sheath

4 Pain on passive extension.

- Treatment involves drainage and irrigation of the flexor sheath.
- This can be performed via an open or closed technique.
- The open technique involves decompressing the finger along its length.
- In the closed technique, the sheath is copiously irrigated through limited proximal and distal incisions.
- A catheter is usually left *in situ* so that irrigation can be carried out post-operatively.

Palm infections

The palm contains three potential spaces deep to the flexor tendons.

The thenar space

- This lies radial to the oblique septum which extends downwards from the palmar fascia to the 3rd metacarpal.
- Flexor sheath infections of the index finger may rupture into this potential space.

The mid-palmar space

- This lies on the ulnar side of the oblique septum.
- Flexor sheath infections of the middle and ring fingers may rupture into this potential space.

The hypothenar space

- This is rarely involved in hand infections.

- These spaces are potential spaces only.
- They are normally empty and only become enlarged in abnormal situations.
- Collections within these spaces should be drained surgically.
- It is important to distinguish between these spaces and the radial and ulnar bursae.
- The radial and ulnar bursae are synovial sheaths which enclose the flexor tendons of the thumb and little finger.
- They communicate proximally at the space of Parona.
- This lies immediately superficial to the pronator quadratus at the wrist.
- Flexor sheath infections of the thumb and little finger can drain through the radial and ulnar bursae into the space of Parona.
- Infection involving both bursae and communicating via the space of Parona is known as a horseshoe abscess.

Dorsal hand infections

The dorsum of the hand contains two spaces.

The dorsal subcutaneous space

- This is a large potential space overlying the entire dorsum of the hand.
- It communicates in the finger webs with the potential space immediately beneath the palmar fascia.
- Palmar infections may spread to the dorsum of the hand via this route.

The dorsal subaponeurotic space

- This space lies just below the extensor retinaculum.
- Drainage can be achieved by incisions:
  1 Over the 2nd metacarpal
  2 Between the 4th and 5th metacarpals.

Further reading

Angrigiani C, Grilli D, Dominikow D *et al.* Posterior interosseous reverse forearm flap: experience with 80 consecutive cases. *Plast Reconstr Surg* 1993; **92** (2): 285–93.

Brand PW. Biomechanics of tendon transfers. *Hand Clin* 1988; **4** (2): 137–54.

Brand PW. Tendon transfers for median and ulnar nerve paralysis. *Orthop Clin North Am* 1970; **1** (2): 447–54.

Brandt K, Khouri RK, Upton J. Free flaps as flow-through vascular conduits for simultaneous coverage and revascularization of the hand or digit. *Plast Reconstr Surg* 1996; **98** (2): 321–7.

Brown DM, Young VL. Hand infections. *South Med J* 1993; **86** (1): 56–66.

Buck-Gramcko D. Pollicization of the index finger. Method and results in aplasia and hypoplasia of the thumb. *J Bone Joint Surg Am* 1971; **53** (8): 1605–17.

Folberg CR, Weiss AP, Akelman E. Cubital tunnel syndrome. Part I: presentation and diagnosis. *Orthop Rev* 1994; **23** (2): 136–44.

Folberg CR, Weiss AP, Akelman E. Cubital tunnel syndrome. Part II: treatment. *Orthop Rev* 1994; **23** (3): 233–41.

Jebson PJ, Engber WD. Radial tunnel syndrome: long-term results of surgical decompression. *J Hand Surg Am* 1997; **22** (5): 889–96.

Mann FA, Wilson AJ, Gilula LA. Radiographic evaluation of the wrist: what does a hand surgeon need to know? *Radiology* 1992; **184** (1): 15–24.

Mayfield JK. Wrist ligamentous anatomy and pathogenesis of carpal instability. *Orthop Clin North Am* 1984; **15** (2): 209–16.

Ninkovic M, Deetjen H, Ohler K *et al.* Emergency free tissue transfer for severe upper extremity injuries. *J Hand Surg* 1995; **20** (1): 53–8.

Olehnik WK, Manske PR, Szerzinski J. Median nerve compression in the proximal forearm. *J Hand Surg* 1994; **19** (1): 121–6.

Quinn MJ, Thompson JE, Crotty K *et al.* Subungual melanoma of the hand. *J Hand Surg Am* 1996; **21** (3): 506–11.

Swanson AB. A classification for congenital limb malformations. *J Hand Surg Am* 1976; **1** (1): 8–22.

Young L, Bartell T, Logan SE. Ganglions of the hand and wrist. *South Med J* 1988; **81** (6): 751–60.

6

The lower limb

Leg ulcers

Leg ulcers are the most common chronic wounds in developed countries.

Aetiology

Leg ulceration may be caused by the following ('VATIMAN').

- **V**enous disease
- **A**rterial disease
- **T**rauma
  - Insect bites
  - Trophic ulcers
  - Self-inflicted injuries
  - Frostbite
  - Radiation
- **I**nfection
  - Bacterial
  - Fungal
  - TB
  - Syphilis
- **M**etabolic disorders
  - Diabetes
  - Necrobiosis lipoidica diabeticorum
  - Pyoderma gangrenosum
  - Porphyria
  - Gout
- **A**utoimmune diseases
  - Lupus
  - Rheumatoid arthritis
  - Polyarteritis nodosa
- **N**eoplasia
  - Squamous cell carcinoma (SCC)—Marjolin's ulcer
  - Basal cell carcinoma (BCC)

- Kaposi's sarcoma
- Lymphoma.

Venous hypertension

- Venous disease is by far the most common cause of lower-limb ulceration and accounts for approximately 80% of cases.
- Venous hypertension usually occurs secondary to valvular incompetence.
- Valvular incompetence usually occurs due to thrombophlebitis.
- Venous hypertension leads to the passage of protein-rich exudate into the subcutaneous tissue.
- This results is lipodermatosclerosis which is characterized by:
  - Scarring
  - Fibrotic, hyperpigmented skin.
- Venous ulcers most commonly occur on the medial aspect of the lower leg.

The leg ulcer patient

Medical history

In patients with leg ulcers, it is important to ascertain the following.

- The time and mechanism by which the ulcer started
- Any previous treatment
- The ambulatory status of the patient
- The type of footwear worn
- The presence of symptoms, such as claudication, that suggest the cause of the ulceration
- Relevant factors in the medical history such as the presence of diabetes.

Examination

During examination particular attention should be paid to the following.

- The ulcer itself
  - The ulcer should be examined for characteristics suggestive of its aetiology.
  - It should also be assessed for any suggestion of malignancy.
- The state of the circulation
  - The temperature of the leg and the state of capillary refill should be assessed.
  - The pulses should be palpated and recorded.
- Sensation
  - Sensation in the lower leg should be assessed.
  - Decreased sensation in a glove-and-stocking distribution is suggestive of diabetic peripheral neuropathy.

Investigation

The following investigations may be indicated in patients with leg ulcers.

- A wound swab
- Measurement of the ankle brachial pressure index (ABPI).
  - This test compares the blood pressure in the arm to that in the leg.

- It is normally in the region of 1.2.
- Decreased readings are suggestive of arterial disease.
- Vascular studies.
  - Venous duplex scanning can be used to assess the venous system.
  - Arterial studies may be indicated in patients suspected of having ischaemic disease.
- Radiography.
  - X-rays and bone scans may be used to assess bony involvement.
- Biopsy.
  - Biopsy should be performed on any long-standing ulcer to exclude the presence of malignancy.

Management

Non-operative

Venous ulcers can be managed non-operatively with:
- Elevation
- Meticulous hygiene
- Elastic compression.

Operative management

- Venous ulceration is not usually managed surgically.
- Indications for surgery include:
  - Intractable pain
  - Failure of non-operative treatment.
- The following operations have been performed for venous ulceration.
  - Subfascial ligation of the perforating vessels
  - Skin grafting—this is associated with a high-recurrence rate, as the underlying venous pathology is not corrected.
  - Excision with flap reconstruction—in exceptional circumstances, fasciocutaneous or free flaps can be used to reconstruct defects after the excision of venous ulcers.

Lower-limb trauma

Incidence

- Over 12 000 open tibial fractures occur in the USA every year.
- Approximately 28% of these fractures are Gustilo 3b injuries.
- Approximately 9% of these fractures are Gustilo 3c injuries.
- Approximately 70% of Gustilo 3b injuries require flap cover.

Classification

- Numerous classifications of lower-limb trauma have been described, including the following.

- The Gustilo and Anderson classification
- The mangled extremity severity score (MESS)
- The AO classification
- The Hidalgo classification
- The Byrd and Spicer classification
- The Arnez and Tyler classification.

- The Gustilo and Anderson and MESS classifications will be described in more detail.

Gustilo and Anderson classification

Lower-limb injuries were originally classified into three grades.

Grade I

- A clean puncture wound <1 cm in diameter
- Minimal muscle contusion
- No crushing injury
- A simple fracture without comminution.

Grade II

- A laceration >1 cm in diameter
- No extensive soft-tissue damage, flaps or avulsions
- A simple fracture without comminution.

Grade III

- Extensive soft-tissue damage, including skin, muscle and neurovascular structures
- High-energy and severe crushing component
- Comminuted fractures
- Segmental fractures
- Bone loss
- Gunshot wounds
- Traumatic amputations.

In 1984, Gustilo further subdivided grade III injuries into the following.

Grade IIIa

- High-energy trauma regardless of the wound size
- Adequate soft-tissue coverage of the bone.

Grade IIIb

- Extensive soft-tissue injury, with periosteal stripping and bone exposure
- Major wound contamination
- Bone loss.

Grade IIIc

An open fracture associated with an arterial injury requiring repair.

Mangled extremity severity score

- The MESS system was designed to assess whether a limb is salvageable.
- A total score of six or less suggests that the limb is salvageable.
- A total score of seven or more suggests that successful salvage of the limb is unlikely.

A Skeletal and soft-tissue injury
Low-energy injury: 1
Medium-energy injury: 2
High-energy injury: 3
Very high-energy injury: 4.

B Limb ischaemia (double the score for ischaemia >6 h)
Pulse reduced or absent, perfusion normal: 1
Pulseless, paraesthetic with diminished capillary refill: 2
Cool, paralysed, insensate or numb: 3.

C The presence of shock
Systolic blood pressure always >90 mmHg: 1
Transient hypotension: 2
Persistent hypotension: 3.

D The age of the patient
<30 years of age: 1
30–50 years of age: 2
>50 years of age: 3.

Management of lower-limb trauma

Mechanism of injury

- It is important to obtain a full history of the accident, as this will provide a guide to the level of energy transferred.
- Factors suggesting high-energy injury include the following.
  - Road traffic accidents
  - Falls from significant heights
  - Missile wounds
  - Any injury involving crushing.

Examination

- Examination will give an indication of the level of energy transferred.
- Factors suggestive of high-energy injury include the following.
  - A large soft-tissue defect
  - A closed degloving injury in which the skin is intact but the perforating vessels are divided
  - The presence of associated injuries

- Segmental injuries
- Imprints from dirt or tyres
- Comminution of bony fragments.

Compartment syndrome

- Compartment syndrome typically occurs after closed leg injuries.
- It can occur in open injuries if:
  1. The compound wound does not extend into the affected compartment.
  2. The compound wound does extend into the affected compartment but has not decompressed it fully.
- Signs of compartment syndrome include:
  - Pain out of proportion to the injury
  - Pain on passive movement of the muscles within the affected compartment
  - A tender or indurated muscle compartment
  - Distal sensory disturbance.
- Absence of peripheral pulses is a late sign and can occur after the muscle compartment has necrosed.
- The presence of pulses does not exclude compartment syndrome.

Measurement of compartment pressures

- Some units monitor compartment pressures in all patients with lower-leg fractures.
- Other units reserve these measurements for clinically suspicious cases.
- If there is any suspicion of compartment syndrome, the compartment pressure should be measured.
- Compartment pressures can be measured via a wick catheter attached to a pressure monitor.
- Pressure monitors are normally used to measure arterial pressure and are available in most operating theatres.
- Ideally, measurements should be taken from all four compartments in the lower leg.
- The deep posterior compartment may be difficult to access.
- The compartment should be decompressed if the pressure within it remains:
  - >30 mmHg
  - <30 mmHg below the diastolic blood pressure.

Fasciotomy of the lower limb

In order not to jeopardize any future flaps, fasciotomy of the lower limb should be performed in the following way.

1 Two vertical incisions are made approximately 2 cm lateral to either side of the subcutaneous border of the tibia.

2 Both posterior compartments are decompressed through the medial of the two incisions.

3 The deep posterior compartment is decompressed by identifying the fascia over the posterior tibial neurovascular bundle at the ankle.

4 This fascia is split upwards, detaching the soleus muscle from its tibial origin.
5 The anterior and peroneal compartments are both decompressed through the lateral incision.
6 The anterior compartment containing the long extensors of the foot lies directly below the lateral incision.
7 The lateral intramuscular septum is divided to decompress the peroneal compartment.

Early surgical management

Patients with severe lower-limb injuries should undergo surgery within 6 h of their injury. The first operation should include:

1 Wound extension
- This allows adequate examination of the soft-tissue and bony injuries.

2 Wound excision
- The skin surrounding the wound should be excised back to bleeding dermis.
- Skin perfusion can be assessed by the administration of intravenous fluorescein.
- A Wood's lamp is then used to detect the presence of fluorescein at the wound edges.
- All necrotic muscle should be removed.
- Muscle viability is assessed by its colour, bleeding pattern and contractility.
- All devitalized or contaminated fragments of bone should be removed.

3 Lavage
- Following debridement, the wound should be irrigated with at least 6 L of fluid.

4 Stabilization of the fracture
- Early fracture stabilization has been shown to reduce morbidity and mortality.
- The fracture should be stabilized with one, or a combination of, the following techniques: (i) intramedullary nailing; (ii) external fixation; and/or (iii) plates.

- A second operation should be performed within 48 h if there is any doubt over the adequacy of the debridement.
- Definitive soft-tissue coverage should be performed within 5 days of the injury.

Soft-tissue coverage

- Wounds requiring flap coverage are usually treated with either:
  - Local fasciocutaneous flaps, or
  - Free-muscle flaps.
- There is some controversy over which is better.
- Proponents of fasciocutaneous flaps maintain that:
  - They are thin and aesthetically superior
  - They may be sensate
  - The operation is quicker and easier to perform.
- Proponents of free-muscle flaps claim that:
  - They conform better to cavities

- Due to their excellent blood supply, they act as so-called muscle macrophages, reducing the likelihood of infection
- With time the muscle thins and provides a good aesthetic result.

Management of bone defects

Bone defects in patients with tibial fractures can be treated in the following ways.

Primary bone shortening

- This technique is often used for segmental defects <5 cm in length.
- Primary bone shortening of defects >5 cm in length may result in the kinking of vessels, resulting in distal ischaemia.

Temporary placement of a bony spacer

- Gentamicin-impregnated methylmethacrylate spacers may be inserted to bridge bony defects and maintain limb length.
- They are subsequently removed and the bony defect is reconstructed by other means.

Bone grafting

- Delayed cancellous-bone grafting is usually performed about 6 weeks after the injury, when the soft tissues have healed.

Primary bone shortening and subsequent lengthening

- Bone lengthening is accomplished by the application of an Ilizarov distraction frame.
- Lengthening at the site of the fracture is known as bone distraction.
- Lengthening at a remote site via a corticotomy is known as bone transport.
- Bone lengthening is usually performed at about 1 mm/day.
- After the desired length has been achieved, the frame is left on for a similar time to the distraction period to allow for consolidation.

Reconstruction with vascularized bone

- Vascularized bone may be used to reconstruct segmental bony defects.
- Vascularized bone can be imported as a free fibula or deep circumflex iliac artery (DCIA) flaps.
- The vascularized bone takes a considerable amount of time to hypertrophy and strengthen.
- During this period, the patient should be strictly non-weight-bearing to minimize the risk of fracture.

Lymphoedema

- Lymphoedema is characterized by the abnormal collection of interstitial fluid.
- It may be caused by maldevelopment of the lymphatics or an acquired obstruction.

The lymphatic system

Anatomy

- Embryonically the lymphatic circulation develops from the venous system.
- Lymphatic channels, unlike blood vessels, do not have well-defined basement membranes.
- Epidermal lymphatic channels do not have valves.
- Dermal lymphatic channels have small valves.
- Muscle has no lymphatic drainage system.
- Lymphoedema is limited to tissue superficial to the deep fascia.
- The superficial lymphatic system drains into the deep system at the following three sites.
  1. Cubital fossa
  2. Popliteal fossa
  3. Inguinal region.
- The deep system of the legs drains into the cysterna chyli.
- This is a thin-walled sac that lies in front of the L1–2 vertebrae.
- The cysterna chyli drains upwards into the thoracic duct at the level of T12.
- The thoracic duct travels upwards alongside the aorta, behind the oesophagus and over the dome of the left pleura.
- It then drains, usually by two or three separate branches, into the left internal jugular vein and the left subclavian vein at their confluence.
- The thoracic duct can be damaged at this point during left-sided, level 4 neck dissections.
- Lymph from the right arm drains into the right subclavian trunk.
- Lymph from the right side of the head and neck drains into the right jugular lymph trunk.

6

Function

- The function of the lymphatic system is to return protein and lipid from the interstitial space to the vascular system.
- 50% of the body's albumin is processed via the lymphatic system every 24 h.
- Lymph is propelled up the lymphatic channels by a combination of:
  - Muscle action
  - Respiratory movement
  - Arterial pulsation.
- Accumulation of lymphatic fluid (lymphoedema) occurs when an increase in lymphatic pressure disrupts the fine valvular mechanism of the lymphatic channels.
- This results in the backflow of lymphatic fluid into the dermis.
- This in turn leads to increased collagen deposition and fibroplasia.
- This fibrosis results in a further increase in the pressure within the lymphatic system.
- As the deep compartments do not have lymphatic channels, lymphoedema is confined to the subcutaneous tissue and the skin.

Classification

Classically, lymphoedema is divided into primary and secondary types.

Primary

- Primary lymphoedema is a diagnosis of exclusion and should only be made when no precipitating cause can be found.
- It is classified by its age of onset into the following types.
- Lymphoedema congenita
  - This is responsible for approximately 20% of all cases of primary lymphoedema.
  - Many affected patients have a positive family history.
  - It is more common in females.
  - 60% of cases occur in the lower limb.
  - 30% of cases are bilateral.
- Lymphoedema praecox
  - This is the most common type of primary lymphoedema, accounting for 70% of cases.
  - Lymphoedema is first noted during puberty.
- Lymphoedema tarda
  - This is the least common type of lymphoedema, accounting for approximately 10% of cases.
  - Lymphoedema becomes apparent after 35 years of age.

Wolfe and Kinmonth have classified primary lymphoedema according to its appearance on lymphangiography into the following types.

- Anaplastic
  - This appearance occurs in 16% of cases of primary lymphoedema.
  - It is characterized by the absence of lymphatics.
  - Anaplastic lymphoedema is usually associated with lymphoedema congenita.
- Hypoplastic
  - This appearance occurs in 67% of cases of primary lymphoedema.
  - Hypoplastic primary lymphoedema can be further subcategorized into:
    - An obstructive form in which a segment of lymphatics is hypoplastic
    - A non-obstructive form in which all the lymphatics are underdeveloped
  - Hypoplastic lymphoedema is usually associated with lymphoedema praecox.
- Hyperplastic
  - This appearance occurs in 17% of cases of primary lymphoedema.
  - It is characterized by an increase in the size and number of lymphatic channels.
  - Hyperplastic lymphoedema is usually associated with lymphoedema tarda.

Secondary

Secondary lymphoedema is classified by its cause. The causes can be remembered as the five 'I's.

1 **I**nvasion by tumour
  - Primary lymphatic tumours
  - Secondary tumours

2 Infection
- The commonest cause of lymphoedema worldwide is filariasis.
- This is caused by the parasite *Wuchereria bancrofti*.
- This can result in massive swelling of the legs and genitalia, known as elephantiasis.
- Lymphogranuloma, TB and recurrent infections are also infective causes of secondary lymphoedema.

3 Inflammation
- Snake bites
- Insect bites

4 Irradiation

5 Iatrogenic causes
- Elective lymph node dissection (ELND)
- Varicose vein stripping.

Clinical diagnosis

- Lymphoedema may be confused clinically with:
  - Lipodystrophy
  - Myxoedema
  - Oedema.
- Simple oedema is distinguished from lymphoedema in the following ways.
  - Lymphoedema is said to be non-pitting.
  - Oedema usually improves within hours of elevation.
  - Lymphoedema improves within days of elevation.
  - Lymphoedematous skin is thick and hyperkeratotic.
  - Secondary lymphoedema usually has factors suggestive of its aetiology in the history.
- Malignant transformation within an area of lymphoedema (lymphangiosarcoma) is said to occur in 10% of severely affected patients after 10 years.
- Stewart–Treves syndrome is malignancy within a lymphoedematous area of the arm, following mastectomy for breast cancer.
- Stewart–Treves syndrome is associated with a high mortality.

Investigation

The following tests may be used to investigate lymphoedema.

Lymphangiography

- In the leg this is performed by injecting patent blue dye into the first web space of the foot.
- The dye is taken up by the lymphatics and helps in their subsequent identification.
- Once identified, the lymph trunks are cannulated and injected with radio-opaque contrast.
- The lymph channels are then imaged radiologically.
- Lymphangiography is seldom used nowadays, as it may worsen the lymphoedema by damaging valves and inducing fibrosis.

6

Interstitial lymphangiography

· In this investigation, contrast material is injected into the interstitial space.
· The contrast is preferentially absorbed by the lymphatic system.
· The anatomy of the lymphatic system is then demonstrated radiologically.

Lymphoscintigraphy

· Antimony (a high-molecular-weight metal) labelled with technetium is injected into the venous system.
· It is preferentially taken up by the lymphatic channels which are imaged radiologically.

CT or MRI scanning

These investigations may be used to demonstrate the architecture of nodal basins.

Non-surgical management

Lymphoedema can be managed non-surgically by the following methods.

Pharmacological treatment

Diethylcarbamazepine

· Diethylcarbamazepine (DEC) can be used to treat filariasis.
· This treatment is effective in reducing lymphoedema in the early stages of the disease, when the worms are small.
· As the worms get bigger, they block the lymphatic channels after they have died.
· Hence, in advanced disease, lymphoedema does not resolve after treatment.

Benzopyrone

· These drugs are coumarin derivatives.
· They bind to interstitial proteins and induce phagocytosis.

Antibiotics

Infection within lymphoedematous areas should be treated aggressively with antibiotics, as it produces fibrosis which can worsen the lymphoedema.

Diuretics

Diuretics should not be used to treat lymphoedema.

Complex decongestive physiotherapy

· This technique was described by Foldi.
· The technique consists of the following phases.
· Phase one—drainage. This involves hospitalization and consists of three parts:

1 Maintenance of hygiene with eradication of fungal infection.

2 Manual lymph drainage, which consists of massage of the normal limb, followed by distal-to-proximal massage of the affected limb.

3 Compressive bandaging and exercise with the limb bandaged.

· Phase two—conservation and optimization. This is performed as an outpatient and consists of elastic support dressings.

Surgical management

Surgical techniques of correcting lymphoedema may be: (i) excisional; or (ii) physiological.

Excisional

Excisional techniques of correcting lymphoedema include the following.

The Charles technique

· This operation involves circumferential excision of lymphoedematous tissue.
· A split-skin graft is then applied to the fascia.
· Resurfacing the fascia with a graft harvested from the excised skin is a later modification of this technique.
· If the skin graft is to be harvested from the excised skin:
  1 A Gibson knife can be used to harvest a thick-skin graft.
  2 The graft is then applied to a glass plate.
  3 The fat is then removed.
  4 The graft is then applied to the fascia.
· The Charles technique is usually reserved for cases with extensive skin involvement.

The Homans technique

· This technique was initially described by Sistrunk in 1918.
· It was later popularized by Homans.
· In this technique, a longitudinal segment of skin and subcutaneous tissue are removed.
· The edges of the incision are then sutured together.
· Surgery usually begins on the medial side of the leg.
· It can be performed on the lateral side as a second procedure.

The Thompson technique

· In this technique, a segment of subcutaneous tissue is excised.
· A dermal flap is then tunnelled through the fascia into a muscular compartment of the leg, in the hope that this might improve lymph drainage.

Liposuction

· This may be useful as an adjunct to other excisional techniques.
· There are concerns that liposuction might induce fibrosis, worsening the lymphoedema.

Physiological

· Physiological surgical techniques aim to improve lymphatic drainage to the limb.

· Numerous operations have been described but, to date, none have proved universally successful.
· Physiological techniques of treating lymphoedema include the following.

Lymphangioplasty

Handley, in 1908, attempted to improve lymphatic drainage by implanting silk threads into subcutaneous tissue.

Omental transfer

In this procedure, a pedicled portion of omentum is transposed to the affected limb.

Enteromesenteric flap

In this procedure, transected iliac or inguinal nodes are covered with a segment of ileum.

Lymphovenous shunts

· This technique anastomoses lymphatic structures to veins.
· It is not suitable in patients with long-standing lymphoedema as they are unlikely to have patent lymphatic channels.

Lympholymphatic anastomosis

· Autologous lymphatic grafts are used to bridge obstructed lymphatic segments.
· This technique may be useful in cases with a short segment of hypoplastic lymphatics.

Pressure sores

· Pressure sores have been observed in bodies found preserved by mummification in Egypt.
· 'Decubitus ulcer' is not an accurate term for pressure sores, as the word 'decubitus' comes from the latin *decumbere*, meaning 'to lie down'.
· Ischial sores usually occur in seated patients.
· Pressure sores develop in approximately 3% of hospitalized patients.
· They are the cause of death in 8% of paraplegic patients.
· Pressure sores tend to occur in:
  · The old
  · The hospitalized
  · The young neurologically impaired.

Anatomical distribution

Pressure sores occur in the following areas in descending order of frequency.

1 Ischium
2 Greater trochanter
3 Sacrum

4 Heel
5 Malleolus
6 Occiput.

Pathogenesis

Pressure sores are initiated by extrinsic factors and propagated by intrinsic factors.

Extrinsic factors

Extrinsic factors include the following.

Pressure

- Pressure causes mechanical damage to tissue, which results in occlusion of vessels.
- If the pressure exceeds the capillary occlusive pressure of 32 mmHg, blood flow within the skin ceases.
- Immobility is an important cause of ulceration, as it results in occlusion of the blood flow for prolonged periods.
- This results in tissue anoxia, which can develop into necrosis and ulceration.

Shear

- This is mechanical stress perpendicular to the surface of the skin.
- It reduces skin perfusion by kinking perforating vessels.

Friction

- Friction is produced by two surfaces moving across each other.
- This results in the loss of the superficial layer of the epidermis.

Intrinsic factors

Intrinsic factors include the following.

General

- Old age
- Malnutrition
- Incontinence of faeces or urine.

Wound

- Local ischaemia or fibrosis
- Decreased sensation
- Loss of autonomic control
- Infection.

Risk scales

Numerous scales have been devised to estimate a patient's risk of developing a pressure sore; they include:

- The Waterlow scale
- The Barden scale
- The Norton scale

Waterlow scale

- The Waterlow pressure-sore risk scale scores the patient's:
  - Build and weight
  - Skin type
  - Continence
  - Mobility
  - Sex and age
  - Appetite.
- Additional points are given for the following specific risk factors.
  - Poor nutrition
  - Sensory disturbances
  - The use of steroids or non-steroidal anti-inflammatory drugs (NSAIDs)
  - Smoking
  - Previous orthopaedic surgery or a fracture below the waist.
- Patients with scores of 10–14 have a risk of developing a pressure sore.
- Patients with scores of 15–19 have a high risk of developing a pressure sore.
- Patients with scores of 20 and above have a very high risk of developing a pressure sore.

Staging

Pressure sores are staged in the following way.

- *Stage 1*
  - Non-blanchable erythema without a breach in the epidermis.
- *Stage 2*
  - Partial-thickness skin loss involving the epidermis and dermis.
- *Stage 3*
  - Full-thickness skin loss extending into the subcutaneous tissue
  - The ulcer does not extend through the underlying fascia.
- *Stage 4*
  - Full-thickness skin loss extending through the underlying fascia
  - Extensive deep destruction
  - Bone, muscle, joint or tendon may be involved.

Prevention

Methods of preventing pressure sores include the following.

- Skin care
  - The skin should be regularly cleaned and dried.
  - Any particulate matter should be removed from beneath the patient.
- Urinary or faecal diversion
  - This should be considered in cases with gross contamination.

- Pressure dispersion
  - Methods of pressure dispersion during sitting or lying may be very effective in preventing pressure sores.
  - The use of low air-loss beds may be necessary in bed-bound patients.
- Pressure awareness
  - Pressure awareness should be taught to all patients at risk of developing pressure sores.
  - Seated patients should lift themselves for 10 s every 10 min.
  - Bed-bound patients should be turned every 2 h.
- Patient positioning
  - Baclofen and diazepam can be used to relieve spasms.
  - Surgical release of contractures, cordotomy or rhizotomy may be indicated to reduce deformity in some patients.

Surgery

Indications for reconstruction

- Patients should be fully investigated before surgery.
- Wherever possible, predisposing factors should be corrected.
- Preventative measures must be in place post-operatively to prevent recurrence.
- Patients with deteriorating conditions are generally not candidates for surgical reconstruction.
- Patients who are expected to increase their mobility are generally treated conservatively as their sores will improve once the pressure is relieved.
- Surgery is best suited to:
  - Well-motivated, young patients
  - Patients with clinically stable conditions
  - Patients who will adhere to post-operative preventative measures.
- Vacuum assisted closure (VAC) can be used as a useful adjunct to speed healing in appropriate cases.

Principles of surgery

The following principles are important in treating pressure sores.

1. An adequate wound excision should be performed; this should include:
   - The surrounding scar
   - Any underlying bursa
   - Bone and soft-tissue calcifications.
2. The resultant dead space should be obliterated.
3. The surface of the defect should be reconstructed with durable skin.
4. Flaps should not be wasted.
   - Flaps that can be readvanced, should the pressure sore recur, should be used whenever possible.
   - If possible, the territories of future potential flaps should not be violated.
5. Flaps should be designed to be as large as possible.

6 Suture lines should lie away from pressure areas.
7 Large drains should be inserted under the flaps and left in place for at least 2 weeks post-operatively.

Reconstruction after excision

Sacral pressure sores

· These defects can be reconstructed with a gluteus maximus musculocutaneous flap.
· This flap can be designed as a rotation flap or a V-to-Y advancement.
· The insertion of the gluteus maximus muscle into the greater trochanter can be divided in non-ambulatory patients.
· This increases the mobility of the flap.
· Lumbosacral flaps can also be used to reconstruct sacral defects.

Ischial pressure sores

· Wherever possible, excision of the ischium should be conservative as complete removal transfers the pressure onto the contralateral ischial process.
· Excision of both ischial processes can result in perineal pressure sores.
· Defects following excision of ischial sores can be reconstructed with V-to-Y flaps based on the hamstring muscles.
  · This flap has the advantage of potential readvancement should the pressure sore recur.
· In ambulatory patients, a posterior (gluteal) thigh flap can be used to reconstruct ischial defects following pressure sore excision.

6

Greater-trochanter pressure sores

· Tensor fascia lata (TFL) flaps can be used to reconstruct defects resulting from excision of these pressure sores.
· They can be designed as V-to-Y advancement or hatchet flaps.
· The designs of both are similar, however the hatchet flap incorporates an intact anterior bridge of skin and deep tissue.

Further reading

Anthony JP, Mathes SJ, Alpert BS. The muscle flap in the treatment of chronic lower extremity osteomyelitis: results in patients over 5 years after treatment. *Plast Reconstr Surg* 1991; **88** (2): 311–8.

Anthony JP, Huntsman WT, Mathes SJ. Changing trends in the management of pelvic pressure ulcers: a 12-year review. *Decubitus* 1992; **5** (3): 44–7, 50–1.

Arnez ZM. Immediate reconstruction of the lower extremity—an update. *Clin Plast Surg* 1991; **18** (3): 449–57.

Choucair MM, Phillips TJ. What is new in clinical research in wound healing. *Dermatol Clin* 1997; **15** (1): 45–58.

Daane S, Poltoratszy P, Rockwell WB. Postmastectomy lymphedema management: evolution of the complex decongestive therapy technique. *Ann Plast Surg* 1998; **40** (2): 128–34.

Eshima I, Mathes SJ, Paty P. Comparison of the intracellular bacterial killing activity of leukocytes in musculocutaneous and random-pattern flaps. *Plast Reconstr Surg* 1990; **86** (3): 541–7.

Foster RD, Anthony JP, Mathes SJ *et al.* Flap selection as a determinant of success in pressure sore coverage. *Arch Surg* 1997; **132** (8): 868–73.

Jamieson WG, DeRose G, Harris KA. Management of venous stasis ulcer: long-term follow up. *Can J Surg* 1990; **33** (3): 222–3.

Klitzman B, Kaalinowski C, Glasofer SL *et al.* Pressure ulcers and pressure relief surfaces. *Clin Plast Surg* 1998; **25** (3): 443–50.

Koshima I, Moriguchi T, Soeda S *et al.* The gluteal perforator based flap for the repair of sacral pressure sores. *Plast Reconstr Surg* 1993; **91** (4): 678–83.

Lai CS, Lin SD, Yang CC *et al.* Limb salvage of infected diabetic foot ulcers with microsurgical free-muscle transfer. *Ann Plast Surg* 1991; **26** (3): 212–20.

Stal S, Serure A, Donovan W *et al.* The perioperative management of the patient with pressure sores. *Ann Plast Surg* 1986; **11** (4): 347–56.

Vasconez HC, Nicholls PJ. Management of extremity injuries with external fixator or Ilizarov devices. Cooperative effort between orthopedic and plastic surgeons. *Clin Plast Surg* 1991; **18** (3): 505–13.

7

The urogenital system

Hypospadias

Definition

- Hypospadias is a congenital condition characterized by:
  - An abnormally proximal position of the urethral meatus on the ventral aspect of the penis or scrotum
  - A hooded prepuce (foreskin)
  - An abnormal fibrous band between the meatus and the glans penis, that may result in ventral curvature of the penis (chordee).
- The following abnormalities may also be present:
  - Paraurethral sinuses
  - Urethral valves
  - A flattened glans penis.

Incidence

- Some degree of hypospadias is present in approximately one in every 300 live male births.
- 50% of cases are associated with inguinal hernias.
- 25% of cases are associated with other abnormalities of the genito-urinary tract.
  - The most common of these is undescended testes, which occur in approximately 15% of patients with hypospadias.
- 4–10% of boys with hypospadias have a positive family history.
- Hypospadias is four times more common in boys born as a result of *in vitro* fertilization.

Aetiology

The following factors have been implicated in the aetiology of hypospadias.

- Androgen-receptor deficiency
- A decrease in the level of epidermal growth factor within the penis during development
- An increase in the levels of exogenous (environmental) oestrogens.

Embryology of the sexual organs

Internal organs

· Prior to the 6th week of gestation, the embryo is sexually indeterminate.

· After the 6th week of gestation, the gonads arise from the genital ridges and differentiate into their male and female forms.

· The internal sexual organs form from the following ducts.

The paramesonephric duct

· This is also known as the Müllerian duct.

· In the female, the Müllerian duct develops into:

1 The fallopian tubes
2 The uterus
3 The cervix
4 The upper part of the vagina.

· In the male, the Müllerian duct degenerates to form the appendix testes.

The mesonephric duct

· This is also known as the Wolffian duct.

· It forms the majority of the internal sexual organs in the male.

· In the male, the Sertoli cells within the gonad secrete a testosterone analogue which acts as a Müllerian-inhibiting factor.

· The Leydig cells of the male gonad secrete testosterone which stimulates the development of:

  · The mesonephric duct
  · The genital tubercle.

· In the male, the mesonephric duct gives rise to:

  · The epididymis
  · The ductus deferens
  · The seminal vesicles
  · The ejaculatory ducts.

External organs

· Prior to the 11th week of gestation, the external genitalia are sexually indistinct.

· At the 11th week of gestation, the external genitalia consist of:

1 A central urethral groove
2 Urethral folds on either side of the urethral groove
3 Labioscrotal swellings on either side of the urethral folds
4 The genital tubercle anteriorly.

In the male

1 The genital tubercle forms the penis.

2 The urethral groove grows distally down the genital tubercle, forming the penile urethra.

- The urethral groove does not quite extend to the tip of the penis.
- The distal part of the urethra is formed by ectodermal ingrowth from the surface of the glans penis.

3 The urethral folds fuse over the urethral groove, forming the tubed urethra.
- The urethral folds fuse in a proximal-to-distal direction.

4 The labioscrotal swellings form the scrotum.
- The testes usually descend into the scrotum at approximately 7 months of gestation.

In the female

1 The genital tubercle forms the clitoris.
2 The urethral groove does not extend into the genital tubercle.
3 The urethral folds do not fuse over the urethral groove. Instead, they form:
- A hood over the clitoris
- The labia minora.

4 The labioscrotal swellings form the labia majora.

Anatomy of the penis

The penis is composed of: (i) the root proximally; (ii) the body in its central portion; and (iii) the glans distally.

The root

The root of the penis is attached to the inferior surface of the perineal membrane. It contains:

- The bulb of the penis centrally
  - This continues as the corpus spongiosum in the body of the penis.
  - The bulb contains the urethra.
- A crus of the penis on each side
  - Each crus continues as the corpus cavernosum in the body of the penis.
  - The deep artery of the penis enters the crus.

The urethra

The urethra is divided into three parts:

1 Prostatic urethra
- This lies within the prostate gland.

2 Membranous urethra
- This passes through the deep perineal pouch.
- It pierces the perineal membrane to become the penile urethra.

3 Penile urethra
- This is also known as the spongy urethra as it lies within the corpus spongiosum.

The tunica albuginea and the fascial layer

- The corpus cavernosum and corpus spongiosum are surrounded and bound to each other by the tough fibres of the tunica albuginea.

· The tunica albuginea is loosely surrounded by the fascia of the penis, which is a cylindrical prolongation of Colles fascia.
· This fascia consists of:
  · The Buck fascia deeply
  · The Dartos fascia superficially.
· Between the tunica albuginea and the loose fascial layer lie:
  · The dorsal artery of the penis
  · The dorsal nerve of the penis
  · The deep dorsal vein of the penis.

Classification
· Hypospadias is classified by the position of the urethral meatus into nine types.
1 Glanular
2 Coronal
3 Subcoronal
4 Distal penile-shaft hypospadias
5 Mid-penile-shaft hypospadias
6 Proximal penile-shaft hypospadias
7 Penoscrotal
8 Scrotal
9 Perineal.

· Glandular, coronal, subcoronal and distal penile-shaft hypospadias are classified as distal and constitute 85% of cases.
· The remainder are classified as proximal and make up the remaining 15% of cases.

Assessment of a child with hypospadias

Important factors in the history
Ask the parents:
· If they have witnessed erections
· Whether they were straight
· Which direction the urinary stream was.

Examination
The examination should include:
· An assessment of the size of the penis
  · If the penis is very small, testosterone cream may be beneficial.
· It is important to check that both testes have descended into the scrotum.
  · If the testes have not descended, genetic analysis should be performed to exclude an intersex state.
· The examiner should exclude the presence of an inguinal hernia.
  · If a hernia is present, investigation of the upper urinary tract may be indicated.
  · This is usually performed by ultrasound examination.

- If possible, the examiner should watch the child pass urine to assess:
  - The direction of the stream
  - The flow.

Surgical correction

Aims and timing of surgery

- Surgical correction of hypospadias should aim to produce:
  - A normal aesthetic appearence including a slit-like terminal meatus
  - Normal erection and sexual function
  - A normal urinary stream.
- Surgical correction of hypospadias is usually performed before 18 months of age.

Techniques

- Surgical correction of hypospadias can be performed as a one- or a two-stage procedure.
- The one-stage procedures can be divided into: (i) urethral advancement techniques; (ii) onlay techniques; and (iii) inlay techniques.

One-stage urethral advancement techniques

Meatal advancement and glanuloplasty incorporated

- This technique is known as the MAGPI procedure.
- It can only be used in cases which have a very distal and mobile meatus.
- The technique involves:
  1. Making a longitudinal incision between the meatus and its intended position
  2. Suturing the longitudinal incision transversely
  3. Advancement of the glans bilaterally around the urethra.

Bulbo-urethral dissection

- In this technique, the whole length of the penile urethra is dissected.
- The technique is also known as bulbar elongation and anastomotic meatoplasty (BEAM).
- The dissected urethra is then advanced until its end lies at the level of a normal meatus.
  - Urethral advancements of up to 5 cm can be achieved.

One-stage onlay techniques

- In these techniques, a patch of vascularized tissue is transposed to form the urethra.
- The patch is not completely tubed as it is in an inlay technique.
- The deep portion of the circumference of the urethra is composed of the intact urethral plate.
- The patch of transposed tissue is sutured to either side of the urethral plate to form a tube.
- One-stage onlay techniques of hypospadias repair include the following.

The Mathieu procedure

This technique is also known as the 'flip-flap'.

1 A distally based skin flap is designed with its base just proximal to the meatus.

2 The flap is then reflected to create the superficial part of the circumference of the urethra.

3 The flap is sutured to the edges of the urethral plate to form a tubed urethra.

4 The gland is then approximated around the neo-urethra.

The onlay island flap technique

In this technique, the superficial part of the circumference of the urethra is reconstructed with a patch of skin from the inner aspect of the prepuce.

1 The flap is pedicled on subcutaneous tissue.

2 It is transposed and sutured to the edges of the urethral plate to form a tubed urethra.

One-stage inlay techniques

These techniques, in which the urethra is reconstructed as a tubed flap, include the following.

The Mustardé repair

- This technique utilizes a similar flap to the Mathieu repair.
- The flap is tubed and used to reconstruct the urethra.

The transverse preputial island flap

This method uses a flap similar to that of the onlay island flap technique.

1 The skin of the flap is designed on the inner surface of the prepuce.

2 It is islanded on a subcutaneous pedicle and tubed to form the neourethra.

Two-stage technique

- This method of hypospadias repair has been popularized by Bracka.
- It is a modification of the original Cloutier operation.

First stage

1 The glans of the penis is split longitudinally.

2 A skin graft is then harvested from the inner surface of the prepuce.

3 The graft is used to resurface the defect.

Second stage

- This is performed approximately 6 months after the first stage.

1 The neo-urethra is formed by tubularizing the skin graft over a catheter.

2 A waterproofing flap of subcutaneous tissue is placed over the suture line.

3 The prepuce can be reconstructed if desired.

- The advantages of the two-stage technique include:
  - Excellent cosmesis with a slit-like terminal meatus
  - Versatility
  - The fact that it can be used for revisional surgery

The technique does, however, have the disadvantage of requiring two operations.

Chordee

- Chordee is longitudinal fibrous tethering on the ventral surface of the penis.
- It may result in bending of the penis on erection.
- If present, chordee should be released during surgery.
- The degree of chordee is assessed intra-operatively with an artificial erection test (Horton test); this is performed by:
  1. Placing a tourniquet around the base of the penis
  2. Injecting sterile saline into one corpus cavernosum.
- Chordee can be corrected by:
  - Simple degloving of the penis
  - Division of the urethral plate
  - Plication of the convex side of the penis (a Nesbit tuck).

Complications of hypospadias surgery

Complications following hypospadias repair can be categorized as follows.

Early complications

- Bladder spasm
- Haematoma
- Wound dehiscence
- Oedema
- Erections
  - These can be suppressed with the anti-androgen cyproterone acetate.

Late complications

- Fistula
- Urethral stenosis
- Persistent urinary tract infections
  - These may occur if hair-bearing skin is used to reconstruct the urethra.
- Balanitis xerotica obliterans (BXO)
  - This condition is also known as lichen sclerosus et atrophicus.
  - It most frequently occurs in the young and old.
  - It presents as a red, ulcerative, sore lesion.
  - These lesions are dysplastic and premalignant.
  - Treatment is by radical excision of the affected skin.
  - The defect can be reconstructed with mucosal grafts from either the mouth or the bladder.
  - Inner preputial skin grafts are not used as they are prone to develop recurrent BXO.

Epispadias and bladder exstrophy

Background

- Epispadias and bladder exstrophy are congenital conditions characterized by the abnormal development of:

- The dorsal surface of the penis
- The abdomen
- The anterior wall of the bladder.

- Exstrophy of the bladder with complete epispadias is the most common deformity and occurs once in every 30 000 live births.
- This deformity is 3–4 times as common in males.
- Epispadias and exstrophy of the bladder are thought to be due to a failure of mesenchymal penetration.

Diagnosis and correction

The clinical features vary from very mild to very major deformities, and may include:

- Epispadias
  - This condition is characterized by a urethra that opens onto the dorsal surface of the penis.
- A cleft clitoris and widely separated labia minora occur in the female.
- Diastasis of the rectus abdominis muscles.
- Absence of the pubic symphysis.
- Exstrophy of the bladder
  - The anterior wall of the bladder may be absent.
  - Eversion of the bladder may occur.
  - Isolated epispadias is repaired with techniques similar to those used for hypospadias.
  - Bladder exstrophy and abdominal wall defects require urinary diversion and reconstruction of the deficient elements.

7

Ambiguous genitalia

- In patients with ambiguous genitalia, it is important to assign the patient's sex before they reach 2 years of age.
- It is crucial that these patients are fully assessed by a geneticist and a paediatrician before this time.
- Ambiguous genitalia occurs in the following syndromes.

Congenital adrenocortical hyperplasia

- This condition is also known as female pseudo-hermaphroditism or adrenogenital syndrome.
- The patients are genetically female (46XX).
- Increased androgen production most commonly occurs due to a deficiency in the enzyme 21-hydroxylase.
- The appearance of the external genitalia varies from a mildly enlarged clitoris to a normal penis with terminal meatus.
- These children should be raised as female and can be fertile.
- Surgical correction may be necessary.
- Surgery is usually performed between 3 and 6 months of age and may include:
  - Clitoral recession
  - Vaginoplasty.

Male pseudo-hermaphroditism

- These patients are genetically male (46XY).
- They have inadequate masculinization of the external genitalia.
- This may be due to:
  - Deficiency in the enzyme 5-α reductase, which results in reduced production of testosterone.
  - Testicular feminization syndrome, which is characterized by the absence of androgen receptors.
- These patients should be raised as female as they would always have an inadequate phallus.
- Surgery involves:
  - Orchidectomy prior to puberty
  - Vaginal reconstruction.

Mixed gonadal dysgenesis

- In this condition, the testis on one side develops normally.
- The other testis does not develop and is known as a 'streak gonad'.
- Most affected children have a 46XY or a 46XO karyotype.
- The normal testis has a high incidence of developing gonadoblastoma.
- These patients should be raised as female.
- Surgery involves:
  - A bilateral gonadectomy
  - Clitoral recession and vaginoplasty.

True hermaphroditism

7

- This condition is very rare.
- Most patients are 46XX.
- Patients may have:
  - An ovary on one side and a testis on the other
  - Bilateral ovotestes.
- These patients should be raised as female as they would always have an inadequate phallus.
- Surgery involves removal of the testis.

Vaginal agenesis

Background

- Vaginal agenesis is known as Mayer–Rokitansky–Küster–Hauser syndrome.
- It occurs approximately once in every 4000 live female births.
- It results from a failure in the development of the paramesonephric duct.
- 50% of cases are associated with abnormalities of the urinary tract.
- The ovaries are usually normal.
- Affected patients sometimes have a vestigial vaginal dimple.
- Cases with no uterus can present with amenorrhoea.

· Patients with vaginal agenesis and a normal uterus may present with haematocolpos.

Investigation

1 External examination
 · This may reveal a vaginal dimple.
2 Ultrasound examination
 · This can be used to define the kidneys, bladder and uterus.
 · It is of limited use in defining the vagina.
3 Intravenous pyelogram (IVP)
 · An IVP should be performed in patients with vaginal agenesis to exclude the high incidence of urinary tract abnormalities.
4 Examination under anaesthesia
 · This can be combined with endoscopy and radiological dye studies to define the extent of the deformity.
5 Chromosomal analysis may be required.

Surgical reconstruction

· Vaginal reconstruction was traditionally delayed until the woman was about to marry in the belief that intercourse would keep the reconstruction patent.
· Nowadays vaginal reconstruction is usually performed during early childhood.
· Many techniques have been used to reconstruct the vagina; they include the following.

Reconstruction with a segment of pedicled colon

This is one of the best methods of vaginal reconstruction.

Dilatation

· This technique was described by Frank in 1938.
· Effective dilatation requires the presence of a vaginal dimple.
· The vagina is sequentially expanded with glass or plastic moulds.

Reconstruction with a split-skin graft

· Vaginal reconstruction with a split-skin graft placed over a mould was described by McIndoe.
· In this technique, the mould is inserted and the labia minora are then oversewn.
· The mould is left *in situ* for 6 months.
· Regular dilatation is required to prevent subsequent stenosis.

Alternative techniques

· The vagina can also be reconstructed with:
 · Full-thickness grafts placed over a stent
 · Flaps of labia minora
 · Regional flaps such as the gracilis.

Further reading

Costa EM, Mendonca BB, Inacio M, *et al.* Management of ambiguous genitalia in pseudohermaphrodites: new perspectives on vaginal dilation. *Fertil Steril* 1997; **67** (2): 229–32.

Duckett JW, Snyder HM III. Meatal advancement and glanduloplasty hypospadias repair after 1,000 cases: avoidance of meatal stenosis and regression. *J Urol* 1992; **147** (3): 665–9.

Johnson D, Coleman DJ. The selective use of a single-stage and a two-stage technique for hypospadias correction in 157 consecutive patients with the aim of normal appearance and function. *Br J Plast Surg* 1998; **51** (3): 195–201.

Newman K, Randolph J, Anderson K. The surgical management of infants and children with ambiguous genitalia: lessons learned from 25 years. *Ann Surg* 1992; **215** (6): 644–53.

Snodgrass W. Tubularized, incised plate urethroplasty for distal hypospadias. *J Urol* 1994; **151** (2): 464–5

Tobin GR, Pursell SH, Day TG Jr. Refinements in vaginal reconstruction using rectus abdominis flaps. *Clin Plast Surg* 1990; **17** (4): 705–12.

Tolhurst DE, van der Helm TW. The treatment of vaginal atresia. *Surg Gynecol Obstet* 1991; **172** (5): 407–14.

Vorstman B, Horton CE, Devine CJ Jr. Current hypospadias techniques. *Ann Plast Surg* 1987; **18** (2): 164–73.

8

Burns

Thermal burns

- Significant thermal burns occur in 0.5% of the population every year.
- Thermal burns tend to occur in:
  - The young
  - The old
  - The unlucky.

Zones of injury

Jackson has classified thermal burns into three zones of injury.

1 An inner zone of coagulative necrosis
2 An intermediate zone of stasis
3 An outer zone of hyperaemia.

Pathophysiology of burn injury

Local effects

- Inflammatory mediators are released from:
  - The capillary wall
  - White blood cells
  - Platelets.
- These inflammatory mediators result in vasodilatation and increased vessel permeability.
- This leads to fluid loss from the circulation into the interstitial space.

Systemic effects

- Systemic effects occur if the burn covers more than 20% of the total body surface area (TBSA).
- The systemic effects of a burn include:
  - Hypovolaemia
  - Immunosuppression
  - Catabolism
  - Loss of the protective function of the gut
  - Pulmonary oedema.

Inhalational injury

Factors suggestive of inhalational injury

Inhalational injury is suggested by the following.

- The history of the incident
  - A fire in an enclosed space
  - The patient lying unconscious in a fire
- Symptoms
  - A hoarse or weak voice
  - Increasing stridor
  - A brassy cough
  - Restlessness
  - Respiratory difficulty
- Signs
  - Soot around the mouth and nose
  - Singed facial and nasal hair
  - A swollen upper airway
  - Hypoxia
  - Pulmonary oedema
  - The development of adult respiratory distress syndrome (ARDS).

Types of inhalational injury

Supraglottic

- This is caused by heat.
- If this injury is suspected, it is imperative to secure the airway before further swelling develops.
- A tracheostomy should be considered in severe cases.

Subglottic

- This is caused by the products of combustion.
- Patients with this injury may require respiratory support, which may consist of:
  - Humidified oxygen
  - Intubation to allow bronchial toilet
  - Intermittent positive pressure ventilation (IPPV).

Systemic

- This may result from the inhalation of carbon monoxide (CO) or cyanide.
- These patients may require respiratory support.

Indications for ventilation

Ventilation should be considered in:

- Patients with a history suggestive of inhalational injury, who have the following signs of respiratory embarrassment:

- A high respiratory rate
- Confusion
- Distress
- Increasing tiredness.

- Patients with extensive burns on the head and neck
- Patients who have supraglottic oedema on fibreoptic examination
- Patients with high levels of carboxyhaemoglobin
- It is imperative that all patients with possible inhalational injury have an anaesthetic review prior to transfer to a burns unit.
- Prophylactic steroids or antibiotics are not indicated in patients with inhalational injuries.

Carbon monoxide poisoning

- CO has 250 times the affinity for haemoglobin as oxygen.
- The half life of CO in patients breathing room air is 250 min.
- The half life of CO in patients breathing 100% oxygen is 40 min.
- CO binds to the intracellular cytochrome system, producing sick cell syndrome.
  - CO levels of 0–15% may be present in smokers or truck drivers.
  - CO levels of 15–20% result in headache and confusion.
  - CO levels of 20–40% result in hallucinations and ataxia.
  - CO levels of 60% are fatal.

Treatment

- CO poisoning should be treated with 100% humidified oxygen, delivered at 8 L/min through a non-rebreathing mask with a reservoir.
- It important to continue 100% oxygen treatment for 48 h following injury, as a secondary release of CO occurs from the cytochrome system.

Referral to a burns unit

The following injuries should be referred to a burns unit.

- Burns covering more than 10% of the total body surface area (TBSA), in adults
- Burns covering more than 5% of the TBSA, in children
- Full-thickness burns covering more than 5% of the BSA, in adults
- Significant burns in the following areas—the hands, the feet, the face, the perineum and over major joints
- Significant electrical or chemical burns
- Any burns in which there is a suspicion of non-accidental injury
- Burns in patients at the extremes of age
- Burns associated with major trauma
- Burns in patients with a significant pre-existing illness.

Estimating burn depth

The depth of a burn can be assessed clinically by its appearance.

	Colour	Capillary refill	Sensation	Blisters	Healing
Superficial	Red	+	+	–	+
Superficial dermal	Pale pink	+	+	Small	+
Mid-dermal	Dark pink	Slow	+	Large	Usually
Deep dermal	Fixed staining	–	–	–	–
Full thickness	White/yellow	–	–	–	–

Estimating the surface area of a burn

The surface area of a burn can be assessed by the following methods.

Comparison with the palm of the hand

- Traditionally, the surface of the patient's hand with fingers adducted has been taken to represent approximately 1% of their TBSA.
- Recent studies have shown that, in fact, this area equates to approximately 0.8% of their TBSA.
- The technique of mapping out the burn with a template of the patient's palm and fingers is a good method of assessing the size of small, patchy burns.

Lund and Browder charts

These charts provide a graphical record of the extent of the burn.

Paediatric Lund and Browder charts

These charts are corrected for the different proportions of a child.

The Wallace rule of nines

- In adults, the surface area of the body is distributed as follows.
  Head and neck: 9%
  Each arm: 9%
  Anterior trunk: 18%
  Posterior trunk: 18%
  Each leg: 18%
  Genitalia: 1%.
- In children, the surface area of the body is distributed as follows.
  Head and neck: 18%
  Each arm: 9%
  Anterior trunk: 18%
  Posterior trunk: 18%
  Each leg: 14%.
- For each year after the age of 10, 1% should be taken off the head and neck measurement and added to the combined legs' measurement.

8

Burn resuscitation

- Fluid resuscitation is required in the following patients.

- Adults with burns (excluding erythema) covering more than 15% of the BSA
- Children with burns (excluding erythema) covering more than 10% of the BSA.

- In most units, fluid resuscitation is administered by one of the following regimes.
  - The Parkland formula
  - The Muir and Barclay formula.
- The Parkland formula gives:
  - 4 mL/kg/% burn of lactated Ringer solution in the first 24 h after the burn.
  - Half of the fluid is given in the first 8 h after injury.
  - The second half of the fluid is given in the next 16 h.
- The Muir and Barclay formula administers fluid in the following aliquots.
  - 0.5 mL^3/kg/% burn of colloid per unit time
  - The time periods are 4 h, 4 h, 4 h, 6 h, 6 h and 12 h.
- It should be emphasized that:
  - These formulas are only estimates of the required amount of fluid; the rate of transfusion should be modified according to clinical parameters.
  - The amount of fluid should be estimated from the time of the burn.
  - These regimens do not include maintenance fluids.
- The urine output during resuscitation should be:
  - >0.5 mL/kg/h in adults
  - >1 mL/kg/h in children.
- The haematocrit should be maintained between:
  - 0.35 and 0.45 in adults
  - 0.28 and 0.35 in children.
- Inhalational injuries and crush injuries require greater amounts of fluid.

Factors specific to children

- Children have reduced physiological reserves and a proportionately greater surface area.
- Because of this, children should receive an additional maintenance infusion of 4% glucose in quarter-strength saline (dextrose saline).
- The volume of this infusion depends on the weight of the child.
  - 100 mL/kg should be given in 24 h for the first 10 kg of the child's weight.
  - 50 mL/kg should be given in 24 h for the next 10 kg of the child's weight.
  - 20 mL/kg should be given in 24 h for the next 10 kg of the child's weight.
- After the initial resuscitation, maintenance fluids should be administered through a nasogastric tube.

Calorific requirements

- The daily calorific requirements are calculated by the Curreri formula:
  - Adults: 25 kcal/kg + 40 kcal/% burn
  - Children: 40–60 kcal/kg.
- The calorie : nitrogen ratio should be 150 : 1.

Timing of surgery

Surgery can be performed in the following periods after burn injury.

Immediate
- Escharotomy
- Tracheostomy.

Early
- Early surgery is performed within 72 h of the burn.
- Early excision and grafting may produce better results than delayed surgery.

Intermediate
- This timing is indicated for patients in whom the burn depth is difficult to determine at the time of injury.
- Many intermediate depth burns, particularly in children, can initially be treated conservatively.
- If they show little sign of healing after 1 week they can be excised and grafted.

Late
- Surgery is classified as late if it occurs more than 3 weeks after the burn.
- Late surgery is seldom indicated.

Burn excision
Burn excision can be performed in the following ways.

Tangential excision
- In this technique, the burn is excised in layers with a skin-graft knife.
- Excision stops when healthy, bleeding tissue is encountered.

Fascial excision
- Burn excision down to the level of the fascia is sometimes indicated in massive burns.
- This technique can be used to limit bleeding in areas in which a tourniquet cannot be used.

Skin grafting

Meshed-skin grafting
- Meshed-skin grafts have the following advantages.
  - The size of the donor site is reduced.
  - Haematoma can escape from under the graft through gaps in the mesh.
  - Meshed grafts contour better than non-meshed grafts.
- The main disadvantage of meshed grafts is their honeycomb appearance when healed.

Full-thickness grafting
- Full-thickness grafts are rarely used as primary cover in acute burns.
- Their main indication is in secondary burns reconstruction.

- Full-thickness grafts have the following advantages over split-skin grafts.
  - They provide a better colour and texture match with the surrounding skin.
  - They contract less.
  - They are more durable.

Non-autograft options for skin coverage

If there are insufficient donor areas for split-skin grafts, the following techniques can be used to cover the excised areas.

Live-related allograft

This is usually harvested from family members.

Live-unrelated allograft

This is freshly harvested at time of organ retrieval.

Cadaveric-unrelated allograft

- This skin may be:
  - Glycerol preserved
  - Cryopreserved at −80 °C.
- Glycerol-preserved skin has a longer lifespan than cryopreserved skin.
- Cryopreserved skin may contain viable cells.
- It may be possible to transmit disease via this route.

Skin substitutes

- A number of skin substitutes are available.
- Some, such as Integra, contain a dermal substitute which becomes integrated into the wound.
- At the present time there is no perfect skin substitute.
- Skin substitutes are used:
  - When insufficient autograft is available
  - As a temporary dressing in a sick patient.

8

The Alexander technique

- This technique utilizes two layers of skin graft.
  - The inner layer is made up of widely meshed autograft.
  - The outer layer is made up of finely meshed allograft.
- This technique is useful in patients with limited donor sites.

The Cuono technique

- In this technique, a biopsy is taken from the unburned skin and sent for cell culture.
- An allograft is then applied as a temporizing measure.
- Approximately 10 days later, the epidermis is removed and the sheet of keratinocytes is applied.
- The dermal element of the allograft may survive, as graft rejection is primarily mediated by Langerhans cells located in the epidermis.

Delayed burn reconstruction

General principles

1 Prevent the formation of contractures, when possible, with exercises and splintage.
2 Give priority to the face and hands.
3 Adhere to aesthetic units whenever possible.
4 Apply sheet grafts to the hands, face and neck.
5 Apply thicker grafts to areas likely to contract, such as the perioral, periorbital and neck regions.
6 Apply pressure garments as soon as possible once the skin is stable.
7 If possible, follow up children until they stop growing.

Treatment of contractures and unstable scars

The surgical options for treating burn contractures and resurfacing areas of unstable scars include:

- Scar revision
- Local flaps, including:
  - Z-plasty
  - W-plasty
  - V-Y plasty
  - Four-flap plasty
  - Five-flap plasty
- Skin grafts (generally reserved for larger areas not amenable for release with local flaps)
- Tissue expansion
- Pedicled or free flaps.

Emergency management of a child with a 40% burn

The emergency management of burns is a common question at all levels of exam; it should include:

8

1 First aid
- Stop the burning process
- Cool the wound

2 Obtain a brief history
- Ascertain the nature and time of the burn
- Ask specifically for factors suggesting inhalational and associated injuries

3 **A**irway management with control of the cervical spine

4 **B**reathing
- Expose the chest
- Assess ventilation
- Administer oxygen

5 **C**irculation
- Control any haemorrhaging
- Monitor the pulse and blood pressure
- Insert two large bore cannulae

6 **D**isability
- Assess the mental status of the patient

7 **E**xposure
- Remove all clothing and exclude other injuries
- Evaluate the TBSA and the depth of the burn
- Assess the need for escharotomies or fasciotomies
- Weigh the patient

8 Resuscitate
- Give a suitable analgesic such as 0.1–0.2 mg morphine per kg
- Administer 100% oxygen
- Take blood for a full blood count, X-matching, urea and electrolytes, carboxyhaemoglobin, glucose and a drug and alcohol screen.
- Start fluid resuscitation according to the Parkland formula
- Take blood gases
- Assess the tetanus status

9 Monitor
- Monitor the pulse, blood pressure and respiratory rate
- Insert a urinary catheter
- Test the urine for the presence of myoglobinuria or haemoglobinuria

10 Once the patient is stable, transfer them to a burns centre after anaesthetic review of the airway.

11 If the TBSA cannot be estimated reliably, resuscitate the patient as a 20% burn. Patients will tolerate this amount of fluid and will not become overloaded, even if no burn exists.

Chemical burns

Chemical burns may be caused by (i) alkalis; (ii) acids; or (iii) other chemicals.

Alkali burns

- Alkali burns cause liquefactive necrosis.
- They often appear less dramatic than acid burns.
- However, they tend to cause deeper injury.
- Alkali burns are commonly caused by:
  - Household bleaches
  - Oven cleaners
  - Fertilizers
  - Cement.

Acid burns

- Acid burns cause coagulative necrosis.
- They should be irrigated within 10 min of injury with:
  - Water
  - Dilute sodium bicarbonate.
- Hydrofluoric acid burns
  - The hydrogen ions cause acid burns.

8

- The free fluoride ions cause extensive local and systemic necrosis.
- Hydrofluoric acid burns should be managed with copious irrigation and repeated application of 10% calcium gluconate.

Phosphorus burns

- Phosphorus is present in:
  - Fireworks
  - Firearms
  - Insecticides
  - Fertilizers.
- Phosphorus burns should be managed with copious irrigation.
- Care must be taken as the phosphorus may re-ignite on drying.

Management of patients with chemical burns

1 Clothing and the causative agent should be removed from the patient.
2 The wounds should be copiously irrigated for up to 1–2 h.
3 Sodium, potassium and lithium burns should not be irrigated with water.
- Water can cause the ignition of these substances.
- These burns should first be extinguished with a fire extinguisher.
- They should then be covered with oil to isolate the metal from any water.

4 The nails, hair and web spaces should be examined for traces of any residual chemical.
5 Ocular injury should be excluded.
6 The local toxicology laboratory may be able to provide information about specific antidotes for particular substances.

Electrical burns

- Current (amps) = voltage/resistance (I = V/R).
- The household voltage is 240 V in the UK and 110 V in the USA.
- The average body resistance is 500 Ω.
- Therefore the current received in an electrical burn from a household plug is:
  - 0.48 A in the UK
  - 0.22 A in the USA.
- Cardiac asystole may result from shocks of 1 A.
- Asystole is more common after a shock with a high-frequency current.

8

Classification of electrical burns

Electrical burns are classified by their voltage.

- Low voltage: <1000 V.
- High voltage: >1000 V.
- Extremely high voltage: lightning strikes.
- Lightning strikes may be:
  - Direct—these are usually fatal.
  - Sideflash—these are caused when lightning strikes a structure such as a tree which then discharges the current through the air or ground to an individual.

· Lightning strikes can cause extensive deep-muscle damage.
· This damage occurs because bone has a high resistance; it therefore heats and causes burning from within.
· Fasciotomies rather than escharotomies may need to be performed in high-voltage injuries, as the deep compartments are often affected.
· Myoglobinuria indicates that muscle is undergoing rhabdomyolysis.
· The resultant deposition of pigment in the renal tubules can lead to acute renal failure.
· Myoglobinuria and haemoglobinurea should be managed by maintaining a high urine output (2 mL/kg/h).
· The urine can be alkalinized with sodium bicarbonate to increase the solubility of the pigments.

Further reading

Arturson MG. The pathophysiology of severe thermal injury. *J Burn Care Rehabil* 1985; **6** (2): 129–46.

Cryer HG, Anigian GM, Miller FB *et al.* Effects of early tangential excision and grafting on survival after burn injury. *Surg Gynecol Obstet* 1991; **173** (6): 449–53.

Demling RH. Burns: fluid and electrolyte management. *Crit Care Clin* 1985; **1** (1): 27–45.

Garner WL, Smith DJ Jr. Reconstruction of burns of the trunk and breast. *Clin Plast Surg* 1992; **19** (3): 683–91.

Heimbach D, Englav L, Grube B *et al.* Burn depth: a review. *World J Surg* 1992; **16** (1): 10–5.

Hunt JL, Sato RM, Baxter CR. Acute electric burns: current diagnostic and therapeutic approaches to management. *Arch Surg* 1980; **115** (4): 434–8.

Neale HW, Kurtzman LC, Goh KB *et al.* Tissue expanders in the lower face and anterior neck in pediatric burn patients: limitations and pitfalls. *Plast Reconstr Surg* 1993; **91** (4): 624–31.

Sobel JB, Goldfarb IW, Slater H *et al.* Inhalation injury: a decade without progress. *J Burn Care Rehabil* 1992; **13** (5): 573–5.

Sykes RA, Mani MM, Hiebert JM. Chemical burns: retrospective review. *J Burn Care Rehabil* 1986; 7 (4): 343–7.

Warden GD. Burn shock resuscitation. *World J Surg* 1992; **16** (1): 16–23.

Microsurgery

History

- Alexis Carrel described the triangulation technique for repair of blood vessels in 1902.
- Malt and McKhann described the first successful arm replantation in 1962.
- Nakayama reported the first series of microsurgical free-tissue transfers in 1964.
- Komatsu and Tamai reported the first successful digital replant in 1968.
- Cobbett performed the first toe-to-hand transfer in 1968.
- Daniel and Taylor and O'Brien and associates independently reported the use of the free-groin flap for leg reconstruction in 1973.

Pathophysiology of vessel healing

Vessel healing following anastomosis

- A thin layer of platelets forms at the anastomosis site immediately after repair.
- These platelet aggregations disappear between 24 and 72 h.
- A pseudo-intima forms at the anastomosis site within 5 days.
- A layer of new endothelium covers the anastomosis site within 1–2 weeks.
- The following factors produce intimal damage and increase the risk of anastomotic thrombosis.

1. Rough vessel dissection
2. Drying out of the vessels
3. Diathermy close to the vessel
4. Prolonged vasospasm
5. Application of a vascular clip with a pressure over 30 g/mm^2
6. The use of large needles
7. Repeated needle stabs
8. Partial thickness suture bites
9. Unequal spacing of sutures
10. Loose sutures
11. Excessively tight sutures

12 Too many sutures
13 High tension across the suture line.

Thrombus formation

- Platelets do not normally adhere to undamaged endothelium.
- Exposure of collagen fibres within the media and adventitia of vessels is a strong trigger for platelet aggregation and degranulation.
- The contents released from the platelet granules include:
  - ADP
  - Thromboxane.
- These substances stimulate further platelet aggregation.
- The intrinsic clotting cascade begins with factor 12 and is initiated by collagen exposure.
- The extrinsic clotting cascade begins with factor 7 and is initiated by tissue factors such as lipoproteins released from damaged cells.
- Both pathways converge at factor 5 and thereafter follow a common pathway.
- The common pathway involves conversion of prothrombin to thrombin, which in turn results in the transformation of fibrinogen to fibrin.
- Fibrin induces the formation of a platelet clump known as a white thrombus.
- As the thrombus grows, the fibrin network ensnares red blood cells becoming a red thrombus.

Drugs limiting thrombus formation

Heparin

- Heparin acts to increase the action of antithrombin 3 which inactivates thrombin.
- This results in a reduction of the conversion of fibrinogen to fibrin.
- The reduced levels of fibrin reduce platelet adhesion.
- A single intravenous dose of heparin may be given at the time of microvascular clamp release.
- Some authorities argue that the subsequent risk of bleeding outweighs any potential benefit.

Dextran

- Dextran is a polysaccharide available in molecular weights of:
  - 40 000 (Dextran 40)
  - 70 000 (Dextran 70).
- Dextran was initially used as a volume expander.
- Subsequently, it was noted to have both antiplatelet and antifibrin properties.
- Animal studies have shown that dextran administration improves anastomotic patency.

Aspirin

- Aspirin inhibits platelet aggregation.
- Its action is mediated by the cyclooxygenase pathway.

Proteolytic enzymes

- The following proteolytic enzymes can be used to dissolve thrombus.
  - Streptokinase
  - Urokinase
  - Tissue plasminogen activator (t-PA).
- Routine administration of anticoagulants or antifibrinolytic agents is not neccesary in uncomplicated free-tissue transfer.
- Some units use dextran routinely in all free-tissue transfers.
- If a post-operative thrombosis occurs, the anastomosis should be explored.
- These patients should probably receive anticoagulant or fibrinolytic therapy.
- In the salvage situation, in which repeated thrombosis of the anastomosis occurs, fibrinolytic therapy should be instituted.

Reperfusion injury

- Reperfusion injury occurs after re-establishment of circulation to a flap.
- Free radicals are substances required for bacterial killing in normal circumstances.
- Free radicals include:
  - The superoxide anion radical O_2
  - The hydroxyl radical OH.
- These two substances combine to produce hydrogen peroxide (H_2O_2).
- An accumulation of free radicals occurs when a flap is devascularized.
- When blood supply to the flap is re-established the following events occur.
  - Endothelial cell damage
  - Endothelial swelling
  - Increased capillary permeability.
- Skin and subcutaneous tissue are relatively tolerant of tissue ischaemia and tolerate:
  - A warm ischaemia time of 6 h
  - A cold ischaemia time of 12 h.
- Muscle is intolerant of ischaemia and develops irreversible changes after:
  - 3 h of warm ischaemia time
  - 8 h of cold ischaemia time.

The no-reflow phenomenon

9

- The no-reflow phenomenon is characterized by failure of tissue perfusion despite adequate arterial input and venous drainage.
- The no-reflow phenomenon is believed to occur due to:
  - Swelling of the vascular endothelium
  - Platelet aggregation
  - Leakage of the intravascular fluid into the interstitial space.
- The no-reflow phenomenon may be treated with:
  - Fibrinolytic drugs
  - Non-steroidal anti-inflammatory drugs (NSAIDs) which act by inhibiting cyclooxygenase.

Equipment

Successful microsurgery requires the following equipment.

Operating microscope or loupes

- Some surgeons prefer to use loupe magnification to repair larger vessels.
- Small vessels are best repaired with the microscope.
- The microscope should ideally be double headed with two ocular sets, so that the surgeon and the assistant can sit opposite each other with the same field of binocular vision.
- The microscope should be able to magnify between ×6 and ×40.
- It should have foot controls for zooming and focusing.
- Ideally, the microscope should have video and photographic attachments.

Instruments

The following instruments should be available on the microsurgical set.

- Four pairs of jeweller's forceps
- Vessel dilators
- Microdissecting scissors
- Needle holders
- Microvascular clamps
  - Single and double microvascular clamps of varying sizes should be available.
  - The clamps should have a closing pressure of less than 30 g/mm^2.

Irrigating solutions

- 100 units/mL of heparin dissolved in Hartmann's solution can be used to irrigate the vessels.
- 5% lidocaine (lignocaine) dissolved in Hartmann's solution can be used to relieve spasm of the vessels.

Sutures

- Monofilament 8, 9, 10 and 11/0 nylon sutures should be available.
- Half-circle atraumatic needles with a diameter of 50–130 μm are normally used.

Technique

Acland described five factors that influence microvascular patency.

1 Surgical precision
2 Diameter of the vessels
3 Blood flow into the anastomosis
4 Tension of the anastomosis
5 Use of anticoagulants or thrombolytic agents.

The following steps are important for successful microvascular transfer.

1 Obtain adequate access.
  - Do not operate down a hole.

2 Operate in a dry field.
3 Position and secure the flap before starting the anastomosis.
- The flap should be tacked into position before starting the anastomosis
- Particular attention should be paid to the pedicle, ensuring it is:
  - The correct length to lie at the anastomosis site without kinking
  - Not twisted or kinked
  - Not compressed.

4 Prepare the vessels for anastomosis.
- Stripping of the adventitia can be performed by gently closing scissors around the pedicle and drawing them distally before cutting the vessel.

5 Flushing the vessel with heparin in Hartmann's solution.
- This should be done gently as excessively powerful irrigation can cause intimal trauma.

6 Limit vessel distension with the dilating forceps.
- Excessive dilation causes spasm of the muscular walls of the vessels.

7 Perform a forward-flow test.
- This should be performed prior to anastomosis.
- In this test, the proximal arterial flow is tested by releasing the clamps on the artery.

8 Never start the anastomosis until you are happy with the set up.
- The following technical points are important during microvascular suturing:
  (i) The needle should be held half-way along its length.
  (ii) The most difficult sutures should generally be inserted first.
  (iii) The needle should be placed in an accessible position within the visual field when tying the knots to facilitate retrieval for the next stitch.
  (iv) Triangulation or bisecting techniques can be used.
  (v) The suture should not be tied if there is any concern that it has caught the posterior wall.
  (vi) After completion of the anastomosis, limit vessel handling as this can result in spasm.

Post-operative management

- The post-operative care of the patient is of paramount importance in ensuring high success rates following microvascular free-tissue transfer.
- Patients should be 'warm, wet and comfortable'.

1 Patients should be nursed in a warm room, and have a warming blanket placed over them during surgery and during transfer.
2 Patients should be well perfused with:
- A urine output of over 1 mL/kg/h
- A systolic blood pressure of over 100 mmHg.

3 The haematocrit should be maintained between 0.25 and 0.35 in adults.
- If it falls below 0.25 blood transfusion should be considered
- If it rises above 0.35 colloid should be given.

4 Patients should be pain free.

Post-operative monitoring

The following techniques can be used to monitor free-tissue transfers in the post-operative period.

Clinical parameters

Those commonly used include:

- Colour
- Temperature
- Tissue turgor
- Capillary return
- Bleeding on pinprick.

Doppler recordings

- This technique is commonly used.
- It can be used to record arterial or venous flow.
- This form of monitoring may give false-positive readings due to sound transmission.

Laser Doppler

- The laser Doppler can be used to:
  - Record blood flow in a small area
  - Scan blood flow over a large area.
- The laser Doppler measures changes in the Doppler shift of light.
- These changes are produced by the movement of macromolecules within vessels.
- The depth of penetration of the laser Doppler is limited to 1.5 mm.

Near infra-red spectroscopy

- This technique is similar to the laser Doppler.
- It utilizes a longer wavelength of light and consequently penetrates deeper.

Temperature measurement

- The temperature of the flap can be measured accurately with a probe.
- A temperature difference greater than 2°C between the flap and the core signifies possible flap ischaemia.
- Differential thermometry is particularly useful for monitoring digital replants.

9

Pulse oximetry

- This technique measures the oxygenation of haemoglobin.
- It is useful for monitoring digital replants.

Impedance monitoring

This technique measures the impedance between two electrodes placed on the flap.

Plethysmography
This technique measures changes in the volume of the flap—increased readings signify flap congestion.

Intravenous fluorescein fusion
- This technique demonstrates blood flow within the flap.
- A test dose of fluorescein is given intravenously.
- This is followed by a dose of 15 mg/kg.
- The passage of fluorescein into the flap can be observed under a Wood's lamp in a darkened room.

Management of non-flowing anastomosis
- This is a common question at all levels of plastic surgical examination.
- The absence of blood-flow through a technically sound anastomosis should be managed in the following way.

1 5% lidocaine should be applied to the anastomosis and a warm, wet gauze placed over it.

2 The anaesthetist should be asked to haemodynamically optimize the patient by ensuring that:
  - They are warm
  - They are well hydrated
  - They are not receiving any vasoconstricting inotropic drugs
  - The blood pressure is raised.

3 Once optimized, the anastomosis should be left undisturbed for at least 15 min.

4 After this time, if the flap is not perfusing adequately, the pedicle should be inspected:
  - Proximally for a twist or compression
  - Distally for a twist or compression.

5 If the anastomosis is not patent or has thrombosed, redo the anastomosis.
  - It is important to avoid excessive manipulation of thrombosed anastomosis as this may send showers of emboli into the flap.

6 If the anastomosis repeatedly thromboses:
  - Consider thrombolytic treatment.
  - Streptokinase can be administered as streptase.
  - 250 000 international units (IUs) of streptase dissolved in normal saline are given as a loading dose over 30 min.
  - This is followed by a maintenance dose of 100 000 IUs per hour.
  - The contraindications to streptokinase treatment include:
    - Administration of steptokinase within the previous 6 months
    - A previous stroke
    - Mitral valve disease
    - The presence of any active bleeding.

Further reading

Cobbett JR. Free digital transfer. Report of a case of transfer of a great toe to replace an amputated thumb. *J Bone Joint Surg* 1969; **51** (4): 677–9.

Goldberg JA, Pederson WC, Barwick WJ. Salvage of free flaps using thrombolytic agents. *J Reconstr Microsurg* 1989; **5** (4): 351–6.

Gordina M. Preferential use of end-to-side arterial anastomosis in free flap transfers. *Plast Reconstr Surg* 1979; **64** (5): 673–82.

Johnson PC, Barker JH. Thrombosis and antithrombotic therapy in microvascular surgery. *Clin Plast Surg* 1992; **19** (4); 799–807.

Jones NF. Intraoperative and postoperative monitoring of microsurgical free tissue transfers. *Clin Plast Surg* 1992; **19** (4): 783–97.

Khouri RK. Avoiding free flap failure. *Clin Plast Surg* 1992; **19** (4): 773–81.

Lister GD, Kalisman M, Tsai TM. Reconstruction of the hand with free microneurovascular toe-to-hand transfer: experience with 54 toe transfers. *Plast Reconstr Surg* 1983; **71** (3): 372–86.

Stassen JM, Lu G, Andreen O *et al.* Intraoperative thrombolytic treatment of microarterial occlusion by selective rt-OA infusion. *Plast Reconstr Surg* 1995; **96** (5): 1215–7.

Strauch B, Greenstein B, Goldstein R *et al.* Problems and complications encountered in replantation surgery. *Hand Clin* 1986; **2** (2): 389–99.

Tamai S. Twenty years' experience of limb replantation—review of 293 upper extremity replants. *J Hand Surg* 1982; 7 (6): 549–56.

10

Aesthetic surgery

With all aesthetic patients, it is important to know:

- What the patient perceives the problem to be
- What their expectations of surgery are
- Why they want the surgery
- Whether they have had any previous, relevant surgery.

Blepharoplasty

- Blepharoplasty is a procedure that is used to shape or modify the appearance of the eyelids.
- It is traditionally performed as the removal of excess skin and fat.
- Recently, several modifications to the traditional technique of blepharoplasty have been described.

Assessment of the patient

Questions

Specific questions for blepharoplasty patients include:

- Whether they wear contact lenses
- Whether they suffer from dry eyes
- Whether they suffer from diplopia.

Examination

The following factors should be assessed during examination of the eyelids.

- The position of the eyebrow
  - Uncompensated brow ptosis is present if the eyebrow is abnormally low at rest.
- Any obvious eyelid pathology
- The amount of excess eyelid tissue
- The position and relative excess of the fat pads
- The presence of lagophthalmos (inability to close the eyelids)
- The position of the eyelids, relative to the eyes

· This is assessed by holding a torch in front of the patient and comparing the distance from the margin of each eyelid to the corneal light reflex.

Tests

After examination of the eyelids, the following tests should be performed.

1 The patient should be examined for compensated brow ptosis.

· Most patients requesting blepharoplasty have some degree of compensated brow ptosis.

· Compensated brow ptosis occurs in patients who have a low eyebrow position with the eyelids closed.

· The presence of compensated brow ptosis is assessed by looking for descent of the eyebrow as the eyelids close.

· When the eyelids are opened, contraction of the frontalis muscle elevates the eyebrow.

· Blepharoplasty alone in patients with compensated brow ptosis may worsen their appearance.

· This is because after upper blepharoplasty the eyelids can open without compensatory elevation of the eyebrow.

· Relaxation of the frontalis muscle causes the eyebrow to descend, which results in a hooded appearance.

· Patients with a significant degree of compensated brow ptosis may benefit from a brow lift prior to, or in conjuction with, a blepharoplasty.

2 The degree of eyelid laxity should be assessed.

· Laxity of the lower eyelid is assessed with the snap test.

· In this test, the lower eyelid is pulled gently downwards towards the cheek.

· On release, the eyelid should rapidly snap back into position.

· Excess laxity of the lower eyelid can be corrected by a horizontal tightening procedure such as a lateral canthopexy.

· This can be performed during blepharoplasty.

3 The location and size of fat pads should be assessed.

· This is performed by gently pushing on the globe and looking for the site and extent of fat herniation.

4 The presence of Bell's phenomenon should be assessed.

· Bell's phenomenon is the protective upward movement of the globe on closure of the eyelids.

· The absence of Bell's phenomenon increases the risk of post-operative corneal exposure.

5 The presence of enophthalmos must be excluded.

· Enophthalmos should be assessed by looking at the position of the globe from above the patient's head.

6 The visual fields should be examined.

· This is often best performed by an ophthalmologist.

7 The visual acuity should be tested and documented.

· The visual acuity should be assessed with and without glasses or contact lenses.

Preoperative counselling

Explanation

- The limitations of surgery should be explained.
  - For example, it is important for the patient to know that the blepharoplasty alone will not improve the appearance of any crow's feet lateral to the orbit.
- The nature of the surgery should be explained. This should include:
  - The type of anaesthesia
  - The incisions and the technique of blepharoplasty
  - The fact that the patient may wake up with eyepads on.
- The post-operative course should be explained. This should include:
  - When the patient can go home
  - What they will look like
  - Any post-operative precautions, such as avoiding straining or leaning over, avoiding non-steroidal anti-inflammatory drugs (NSAIDs), and the application of damp pads to the eyes at night
  - The arrangements for follow-up.

Possible complications

- It is important to discuss possible complications. These should be divided into:
  - Intra-operative complications
  - Early complications
  - Late complications.
- It is important to mention the risk of blindness, although it should be emphasized that it is extremely rare.
  - Post-operative blindness is usually caused by a retrobulbar haematoma (a haematoma behind the orbital septum).
  - Once identified, this is a surgical emergency and should be managed with orbital decompression by release of the septum or lateral canthus.
  - The carbonic anhydrase inhibitor acetazolamide and mannitol should then be administered in an effort to further decompress the orbit pharmaceutically.

Techniques of blepharoplasty

The traditional technique

Upper-eyelid blepharoplasty

- The patient is placed in a supine position with their head up.
- The lower border of the skin excision is defined.
- The upper border of the skin excision is assessed by gently pinching the eyelid skin between the blades of a pair of blunt forceps.
- The upper border of the skin excision is defined at multiple points across the upper eyelid.
- A strip of skin and the underlying orbicularis oculi muscle is then removed from between the upper and lower borders of the skin excision.

- The fat pads are accessed though small incisions in the orbital septum.
- A clip is placed across the base of the fat pads and they are transected.
- Light diathermy is applied to the transected base of the fat pad.

Lower-eyelid blepharoplasty

- An incision is made just below the eyelash margin.
- This incision is extended laterally along a natural skin crease.
- The lower-eyelid skin can be elevated alone or with a strip of the underlying orbicularis oculi muscle.
- The three lower-eyelid fat pads are accessed though small incisions in the orbital septum.
- Excess fat is removed in the same way as in the upper eyelid.
- The lower-eyelid skin is then redraped and the amount of excess tissue is assessed.
- The excess skin is excised and the wound is closed with fine sutures.

Variations on the traditional technique

Limited fat removal from the lower eyelid

- Some authorities contend that the removal of fat from the lower eyelid can result in a sunken appearance.
- The grooves at the junction of the eyelid and cheek skin are known as tear-trough deformities.
- Correction of the tear-trough deformity can be performed by:
  - Transposing pedicles of orbital fat into these areas
  - Inserting a Flower's tear-trough implant

Brow lifting

Brow lifting, either by an open or endoscopic technique, should be considered if the patient has significant compensated or uncompensated brow ptosis.

Upper-eyelid skin invaginating procedures

- The upper-eyelid fold can be reconstructed during blepharoplasty.
- This is performed by tacking the superficial layers of the upper eyelid to the deeper structures.

Lower-eyelid transconjunctival blepharoplasty

- Excess fat within the lower eyelid can be removed via a transconjunctival approach.
- In this procedure, the fat pads are accessed though an incision on the inner surface of the eyelid.
- This approach avoids external scarring.
- Redundant eyelid skin cannot be excised by this method.
- However, lasers and chemical peels can be used to tighten the lower eyelid.

Lower-lid tightening procedures

Tightening the lower eyelid can be performed with:

- A lateral canthopexy
- A wedge resection
  - Wedge resection of the lower eyelid can result in notching of the eyelid margin.
  - The use of wedge resections is often reserved for patients with ectropion.

Face lifting

Anatomy

The superficial musculoaponeurotic system

- The superficial musculoaponeurotic system (SMAS) is a layer of facial fascia.
- The SMAS is contiguous with the:
  - Frontalis muscle
  - Galea aponeurotica
  - Temporoparietal fascia (superficial temporal fascia)
  - Platysma muscle.
- These structures form a continuous layer of superficial fascia in the forehead, temple, face and neck.
- The SMAS is tightly adherent to the zygomatic arch.
- It becomes less distinct anteriorly at the level of the nasolabial crease.
- Sensory nerves tend to lie superficial to the SMAS.
- Motor branches of the facial nerve tend to lie deep to the SMAS.

The retaining ligaments of the face

The skin of the face is secured to the underlying muscles and bone by the following retaining ligaments.

- Osseocutaneous ligaments
  - These ligaments pass from the bone to the skin.
  - They occur over the zygoma (McGregor's patch) and over the anterior part of the mandible.
- Musculocutaneous ligaments
  - These are condensations between the underlying muscle fascia and the skin.
  - They occur between the parotid fascia and the skin (parotid-cutaneous ligaments) and the masseter muscle and the skin (masseteric-cutaneous ligaments).

The frontal branch of the facial nerve

- This branch of the facial nerve is unusual in that it becomes relatively superficial as it travels distally.
- It runs along Pitanguy's line, which passes from 0.5 cm below the tragus to 1.5 cm above and lateral to the eyebrow.
- The nerve becomes more superficial superiorly, and lies just under the temporoparietal fascia in the temple.

The greater auricular nerve

- This is a branch of the cervical plexus.
- It emerges from behind the sternocleidomastoid, approximately 6.5 cm below the tragus.
- Care should be taken to preserve this nerve during face-lift procedures, as it supplies sensation to the inner and outer aspects of the lower half of the ear.

Assessment of the patient

Questions

Specific questions for patients considering a face lift include:

- Whether they smoke
- Whether they have high blood pressure
- Whether they are on any relevant medication, such as aspirin
- Whether there are any relevant factors in their medical history, such as healing disorders, diabetes or rheumatoid arthritis.

Examination

The following factors should be assessed during examination:

- Distribution of excess tissue
- Distribution of wrinkling
- Quality of the skin
- Facial asymmetry
- Facial power
- Position of the earlobes
- Condition of the hair, because if there is hair loss preoperatively the risk of alopecia after surgery is increased
- The best vector in which to tighten the face.

Techniques

Skin-only face lift

- This involves subcutaneous undermining of the skin on the cheek and neck.
- Dissection can extend as far medially as the nasolabial crease.
- This type of face lift may be subject to early recurrence as the underlying structures are not tightened.

Skin-and-SMAS face lift

- In this type of face lift, the skin of the cheek is undermined as in a skin-only face lift.
- The SMAS layer is then dissected as a separate flap.
- The extent of the dissection under the SMAS varies and may proceed as far medially as the nasolabial crease.
- The zygomatic and masseteric restraining ligaments are released to increase the mobility of the SMAS flap.
- The dissected SMAS layer is tightened and secured anterior to the ear.
- The excess SMAS can be used to augment the zygomatic arch.

Deep-plane face lift

- In this operation, dissection of the cheek is performed under the SMAS layer.
- The layer between the SMAS and the skin is not dissected.
- The composite flap of cheek skin and SMAS is then tightened and secured.
- This form of face lift may be indicated in heavy smokers, as the undermined cheek and SMAS flap is thicker and less prone to necrosis.

Mid-face suspension

- In this procedure, the deep tissues of the mid-face are dissected through a lower blepharoplasty or temporal incision.
- A suture is placed through the soft tissue of the cheek and passed up to the temple.
- The mid-face is elevated by tightening the suture and securing it to the superficial layer of the deep temporal fascia.

Non-endoscopic, subperiosteal face lift

In this procedure, the soft tissues of the face are dissected in a subperiosteal plane through a number of open incisions.

Endoscopic face lift

- In this procedure, the face is dissected endoscopically at a subperiosteal level.
- Once freed from its bony attachments, the face can be elevated and secured.
- This form of face lift is usually performed on younger patients without significant amounts of excess skin.

Management of the neck

- Divarication of the platysma muscles can produce unsightly bands at their medial borders.
- The appearance of the neck can be improved by:
  - Submental defatting
  - Plication of the medial borders of the platysma muscle to one another
  - Resection or division of the prominent platysmal bands.
- Laser resurfacing can be performed at the same time as the face lift.
- Laser resurfacing is generally not performed on undermined skin flaps as this may increase the risk of necrosis and delayed healing.

Possible complications

The possible complications following face lifting include:

- Haematoma
- Skin necrosis
- Nerve injury
- Alopecia
- Excessive scarring
- Changes in skin pigmentation.

Rhinoplasty

Anatomy

Skeleton

The skeleton of the nose can be divided into thirds.

Upper-third

The upper-third of the nasal skeleton consists of paired nasal bones which interdigitate with:

- The nasal process of the frontal bone superiorly
- The frontal process of the maxilla laterally.

Middle-third

The middle-third of the nasal skeleton consists of paired upper-lateral cartilages.

- The upper-lateral cartilages are fused to the undersurface of the nasal bones superiorly.
- The lower (caudal) edge of the upper-lateral cartilages lie under the upper (cephalad) border of the lower-lateral cartilages.
- The inferior end of the upper-lateral cartilage forms the internal nasal valve.

Lower-third

The lower-third of the nose consists of paired alar (also called lower-lateral) cartilages.

- These are curved structures which meet at their apex to form the tip of the nose.
- Each alar cartilage is composed of:
  - A medial crus, which runs through the columella
  - A middle crus, which forms the nasal tip
  - A lateral crus, which passes upwards and outwards from the nasal tip.
- The alar cartilages do not curve laterally along the alar margins but incline upwards and outwards in an oblique direction.
- At their upper border they overlie the cephalad portion of the upper-lateral cartilages.

Septum

- The nasal septum is composed of:
  - The quadrangular cartilage anteriorly
  - The perpendicular plate of the ethmoid superiorly
  - The vomer inferiorly.
- A small part of the inferior margin of the nasal septum is made up of:
  - The perpendicular process of the maxilla anteriorly
  - The perpendicular plate of the palatine bone posteriorly.
- The membranous septum is at the caudal end of the cartilaginous septum.
- It connects the cartilaginous septum to the medial crura of the alar cartilages.
- A transfixing incision passes through the membranous septum.

Specific terms

The following terms may be used when discussing rhinoplasty.

- The tip-defining points are the most prominent areas of the nasal tip.
- Nasal length is the distance from the nasofrontal groove to the nasal tip.
- Tip projection is the distance from the nasal spine to the nasal tip.
- The bony vault is the area overlying the nasal bones.
- The cartilaginous vault is the area overlying the upper-lateral cartilages.
- The lobule is the area overlying the alar cartilages.
- The supratip is just above the domes of the alar cartilages.
- The soft triangle is a small area of the rim of the nose that does not contain cartilage; it lies between the nasal rim and the lower border of the dome of the alar cartilage.
- The infratip lobule extends from the nasal tip to the start of the columella.
- An open roof is the appearance of the nasal dorsum after dorsal hump removal and prior to in-fracture.
- An out-fracture is a manoeuvre that mobilizes the nasal bones prior to their subsequent in-fracture.
- An in-fracture is the medial movement of the nasal bones necessary to correct the open roof deformity.

Assessment of the patient

Questions

Specific questions for rhinoplasty patients include:

- Whether they have any problems breathing through their nose
- Whether they suffer from nosebleeds
- Whether they suffer from allergic rhinitis
- Whether they suffer from regular headaches
- Whether their profession depends on a sense of smell (e.g. wine tasters)
- Whether they have ever taken drugs nasally (e.g. cocaine).

Examination

The following facial factors should be assessed when examining the nose.

- The overall shape of the face
- The proportions of the underlying skeleton
- Dental occlusion
- The thickness of the nasal skin
- The nasal angles and proportions
- The form of the nasal tip
- The nasal septum and turbinates
    - Intranasal examinations should be performed.
- The presence of nasal valving
- The presence of the 'Cottle sign'
    - The 'Cottle sign' is present when lateral cheek traction opens the nasal valve and improves air entry into the nose.

Techniques

- Some authors recommend nasal packing preoperatively with swabs soaked in 5% cocaine or Moffett's solution, in an effort to reduce intra-operative bleeding.
- The nose is usually infiltrated with local anaesthetic containing epinephrine (adrenaline).
- Rhinoplasty can be performed through:
  - A closed (endonasal) approach—this technique is longer established and more commonly performed.
  - An open approach—this may be preferred in patients requiring a significant amount of surgery on the nasal tip.

Types of incision

The following incisions are used to access the internal structure of the nose.

Rim incision

- This incision lies just inside the rim of the nose.
- It is used as a continuation of the transcolumella incision, to expose the internal structure of the nose during open rhinoplasty.

Transcartilaginous incision

- This is also known as an intracartilaginous incision.
- It is used during closed rhinoplasty to gain access to the dorsum of the nose.
- The incision passes through the lining of the nose and the alar cartilage.
- The portion of alar cartilage above the incision is removed while the portion below is preserved.

Intercartilaginous incision

- This is an alternative to the transcartilaginous incision.
- The incision passes between the alar cartilage and the upper lateral cartilage.
- The upper part of the alar cartilage can be removed as a secondary step.

Transfixion incision

- This passes through the membranous septum, between the cartilaginous septum above and the medial crura of the alar cartilages below.

Alar base excision

Resections of the alar base are used to reduce the width of the nose.

Osteotomies

- Resection of the dorsum of the nose can be performed with an osteotome or rasp.
- This results in an open roof deformity which needs to be corrected by an in-fracture of the nasal bones.
- To perform an in-fracture the nasal bones need to be weakened at their bases by an osteotomy.

· Osteotomies of the nasal bones can be performed:
  · With fine osteotomes (or saws) inserted along their outer surface through small intranasal incisions
  · Transcutaneously with a fine osteotome.

Osteotomies of the nasal bones may be:

Low-to-high

· These start low at the junction of the nose and the cheek.
· They end just below the medial canthus, above the junction of the nose and the cheek.
· They do not usually require an additional percutaneous osteotomy to mobilize the nasal bones.

Low-to-low

· These osteotomies are sometimes indicated in male patients with broad noses.
· They start at the same site as the low-to-high osteotomies.
· They end just below the medial canthus closer to the cheek than the low-to-high osteotomies

Some authors perform an additional transverse percutaneous osteotomy, close to the medial canthus, to mobilize the nasal bones prior to their in-fracture.

Correction of the nasal tip

· Correction of the nasal tip can be performed by:
  · Insertion of cartilage grafts
  · Suture techniques
· There is considerable debate as to which technique provides the best results.

Grafts

Several types of grafts can be used in rhinoplasty; they include:

· Tip grafts
  · These can be simple, shield-like onlay grafts.
  · They can include a strut, which is inserted down the columella between the medial crura of the alar cartilages.
  · This type of graft is called an umbrella graft.
· Spreader grafts
  · These matchstick-like cartilage grafts are used to widen the middle third of the nose, and to correct nasal valving.
  · They are placed between the nasal septum and the upper-lateral cartilages.
  · They prevent collapse of the upper-lateral cartilages at the internal nasal valve on inspiration.

Suture techniques

· Suture techniques are principally used to modify the shape of the alar cartilages in the nasal tip.
· Autoclavable models of 'ideal alar cartilages' are available to aid intra-operative shaping of the cartilages during open rhinoplasty.
· A number of tip-suturing techniques have been described.

- Sutures can be placed:
  - Between the medial crura of each alar cartilage, to stabilize and narrow the columella
  - Between the medial and lateral crura of each alar cartilage, to accentuate the curvature of their domes
  - Between the domes of the alar cartilages, to bring them together and narrow the tip of the nose
  - Between the membranous part of the nasal septum and the medial crura of the alar cartilage, to increase or decrease tip projection.

Liposuction

Anatomy

- Subcutaneous fat is divided by the superficial fascia into superficial and deep compartments.
- The superficial compartment contains densely packed fibrous stroma arranged vertically and horizontally.
- This compact structure is responsible for the skin dimpling seen in patients described as having 'cellulite'.
- The deep compartment contains much less compact fibrous stroma.
- The number of fat cells in an individual does not increase after puberty.
- Once fat cells have been removed, they will not come back.
- The remaining cells can, however, hypertrophy.
- Men deposit fat in an android pattern around the abdomen and torso.
- Women deposit fat in a gynaecoid pattern around the hips and thighs.

Techniques

Liposuction can be performed using the following techniques.

Dry liposuction

- This was the original method of liposuction.
- This technique may be associated with a high blood loss as no infiltrate is used.

Wet liposuction

In this technique, 200–400 mL of infiltrate is infused per area.

Superwet liposuction

This technique aims to infuse 1 mL of infiltrate for every mL of fat aspirated.

The tumescent technique

- This technique aims to infuse 2–3 mL of infiltrate for every mL of fat aspirated.
- The composition of the infiltrate varies between surgeons.
- A commonly used recipe for the infiltrate is:
  1. 25 mL of 2% lidocaine (xylocaine)
  2. 1 mL of 1 : 1000 epinephrine
  3. 1000 mL of warmed lactated Ringer solution.

- This produces a concentration of:
  - 0.05% lidocaine
  - 1 : 1 000 000 epinephrine.
- Some authors prefer to use NaCl rather than Hartmann's solution as it contains less potassium.
- Some authors maintain that the local anaesthetic within the infiltrate can be used as the sole means of anaesthesia.
- The advantages of the tumescent technique include less blood loss and post-operative analgesia.
- However, large volumes of infiltrate can result in disturbances in fluid balance.

Ultrasonic-assisted liposuction

- In this technique, ultrasonic energy, delivered by a probe, is used to liquefy fat cells.
- This process is known as cavitation.
- The liquefied fat is then removed in a similar fashion to traditional liposuction.
- This technique has the following advantages.
  - It may be more effective at removing fat in conditions such as gynaecomastia.
  - It significantly reduces the operator fatigue associated with liposuction.
- There are concerns that the heat generated by the ultrasonic probe may cause soft-tissue burns.

Power-assisted liposuction

- Recently, power-assisted cannulas have been developed.
- These non-ultrasonic devices are said to maximize fat removal while reducing the effort required during liposuction.

Possible complications

The possible complications of liposuction include:

- Contour irregularities can occur particularly if the liposuction was performed too superficially or excessively at one site.
- Damage to adjacent structures.
- Paraesthesia.
- Haemorrhage.
- Fluid shifts.
- Death.
  - There have been reports of deaths following liposuction (*N Engl J Med* 1999; 340:1471–5).
  - Three of four of these deaths was attributed to pulmonary embolism rather than excess fluid injection during the tumescent technique.

Further reading

De la Plaza R, Arroyo JM. A new technique for the treatment of palpebral bags. *Plast Reconstr Surg* 1988; **81** (5): 677–87.

Hamra ST. Arcus marginalis release and orbital fat preservation in midface rejuveination. *Plast Reconstr Surg* 1995; **96** (2): 354–62.

Hamra ST. The deep-plane rhytidectomy. *Plast Reconstr Surg* 1990; **86** (1): 53–61.

Hamra ST. Composite rhytidectomy and the nasolabial fold. *Clin Plast Surg* 1995; **22** (2): 313–24.

Har-Shai Y, Bodner SR, Egozy-Golan D *et al.* Mechanical properties and microstructure of the superficial musculo-aponeurotic system. *Plast Reconstr Surg* 1996; **98** (1): 59–70.

Jelks GW, Jelks EB. Preoperative evaluation of the blepharoplasty patient: bypassing the pitfalls. *Clin Plast Surg* 1993; **20** (2): 213–23.

Lockwood T. High-lateral-tension abdominoplasty with superficial fascial system suspension. *Plast Reconstr Surg* 1995; **96** (3): 603–15.

Lockwood T. Lower body lift with superficial fascial system suspension. *Plast Reconstr Surg* 1993; **92** (6): 1112–22.

Lockwood T. The role of excisional lifting in body contour surgery. *Clin Plast Surg* 1996; **23** (4): 695–712.

Maxwell CP, Gingrass MK. Ultrasound-assisted lipoplasty: a clinical study of 250 consecutive patients. *Plast Reconstr Surg* 1998; **101** (1): 189–202.

Rohrich RJ, Beran SJ, Fodor PB. The role of subcutaneous infiltration in suction-assisted lipoplasty: a review. *Plast Reconstr Surg* 1997; **99** (2): 514–9.

Rudolph R. Depth of the facial nerve in face lift dissections. *Plast Reconstr Surg* 1990; **85** (4): 537–44.

Sheen JH. Rhinoplasty: personal evolution and milestones. *Plast Reconstr Surg* 2000; **105** (5): 1820–52.

Tebbetts JB. Blepharoplasty: a refined technique emphasizing accuracy and control. *Clin Plast Surg* 1992; **19** (2): 329–49.

Zarem HA, Resnick JI. Operative technique for transconjunctival lower blepharoplasty. *Clin Plast Surg* 1992; **19** (2): 351–6.

Index